Sociology and Occupational Therapy

For Churchill Livingstone

Editorial Director: Mary Law
Project Manager: Valerie Burgess
Project Editor: Valerie Dearing
Copy Editor: Carrie Walker
Indexer: Liz Grainger
Design Direction: Judith Wright
Sales Promotion Executive: Hilary Brown

Sociology and Occupational Therapy

An Integrated Approach

Edited by

Derek Jones BA(Hons) DipCOT SROT
Lecturer in Occupational Therapy, Department of Occupational Therapy
and Art Therapy, Queen Margaret College, Leith Campus, Edinburgh UK

Sheena E. E. Blair MEd DipCOT SROT
Senior Lecturer and Course Leader, Department of Occupational Therapy
and Art Therapy, Queen Margaret College, Leith Campus, Edinburgh UK

Terry Hartery BSc(Hons) MSocSc
Lecturer in Sociology, Department of Management and Social Sciences,
Queen Margaret College, Edinburgh UK

R. Kenneth Jones BA(Hons) Cert Rel Stud ACE PhD FCollP FRSA
Lecturer in Health and Illness, Department of Management and Social Sciences,
Queen Margaret College, Edinburgh UK

Foreword by

Elizabeth Townsend Phd OT(C) RegNS
Associate Professor and Director, School of Occupational Therapy,
Dalhousie University, Halifax, Nova Scotia, Canada

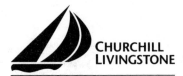

EDINBURGH LONDON NEW YORK PHILADELPHIA SYDNEY TORONTO TOKYO 1998

CHURCHILL LIVINGSTONE
An imprint of Harcourt Brace and Company Limited

First published 1998

ISBN 0 443 055157

British Library Cataloguing in Publication Data
A catalogue record for this book is available from the British
Library.

Library of Congress Cataloging in Publication Data
A catalog record for this book is available from the Library
of Congress.

The
publisher's
policy is to use
**paper manufactured
from sustainable forests**

Produced by Addison Wesley Longman China Limited, Hong Kong
GCC/01

Contents

Contributors

Sheena E. E. Blair MEd Dip COT SROT
Senior Lecturer and Course Leader, Department
of Occupational Therapy and Art Therapy,
Queen Margaret College, Leith Campus,
Edinburgh, UK

Anita C. Bundy ScD OTR FAOTA
Associate Professor, Colorado State University,
Department of Occupational Therapy,
Fort Collins, Colorado, USA

Isabel Dyck DipOT BA MA PhD
Associate Professor, School of Rehabilitation
Sciences, University of British Columbia,
Canada

Thomas Gahagan BSc(Hons) SROT
Community Occupational Therapist, Edinburgh
City Council Social Work Department,
Edinburgh, UK

Terry Hartery BSc(Hons) MSocSc
Lecturer in Sociology, Department of
Management and Social Sciences,
Queen Margaret College, Edinburgh, UK

Chris Jones BA(Hons) MSc DipCOT
Project Manager, SHS Ltd, Edinburgh, UK

Derek Jones BA(Hons) Dip COT SROT
Lecturer in Occupational Therapy, Department
of Occupational Therapy and Art Therapy,
Queen Margaret College, Leith Campus,
Edinburgh, UK

R. Kenneth Jones BA(Hons) Cert Rel Stud ACE PhD
FCollP FRSA
Lecturer in Health and Illness, Department of
Management and Social Sciences,
Queen Margaret College, Edinburgh, UK

Carol Lennie BA(Hons)
Tutor, Open University and Lecturer,
Department of Government, University of
Strathclyde, Glasgow, UK

Doreen E. MacWhannell MPhil MSc MCSP CertEd ONC
Senior Lecturer, Department of Management
and Social Sciences, Queen Margaret College,
Edinburgh, UK

Ian R. McMillan MEd DipCOT CertEd(FE) SROT
Lecturer in Occupational Therapy, Department
of Occupational Therapy and Art Therapy,
Queen Margaret College, Leith Campus,
Edinburgh, UK

M. Margaret Nicol Phd MPhil DipCOT
Senior Lecturer in Occupational Therapy,
Department of Occupational Therapy and Art
Therapy, Queen Margaret College, Leith
Campus, Edinburgh, UK

Christine Ravetz DipCOT SROT BA(Hons) MA
Head of Department, Centre for Occupational
Therapy Education, School of Health,
St Martins College, Lancaster, UK

Linda Renton BSc(Hons) DipCOT SROT
Lecturer in Occupational Therapy, Department
of Occupational Therapy and Art Therapy,
Queen Margaret College, Leith Campus,
Edinburgh, UK

Kristen Stalker BA PhD CQSW
Senior Research Fellow, Social Work Research
Centre, University of Stirling, UK

Averil Stewart BA FCOT TDipSROT
Professor and Head of Department of
Occupational Therapy and Art Therapy, Queen
Margaret College, Leith Campus, Edinburgh, UK

Louise R, Thibodaux MA OTR FAOTA
Associate Professor, University of Alabama at
Birmingham, Division of Occupational
Therapy, Birmingham, Alabama, USA

Chris Yuill MA(Hons) PG DipLib&InfoTech
Lecturer in Sociology, Robert Gordon
University, Aberdeen, UK

Foreword

I discovered sociology after 20 years of practice as an occupational therapist. Studying sociology as a graduate student helped me to make sense of my experiences with people whose lives were made easier or more difficult by what occupational therapists now describe as the clients' environment: physical access to buildings; availability of family and monetary support for living at home; cultural attitudes to people with a mental illness who try to hold a job; policies regarding school-based services for children with disabilities. Furthermore, sociology offered me theories and methods for understanding the context of my occupational therapy practice in settings as diverse as hospitals, rehabilitation centres, health and mental health clinics, schools, homes, workplaces, and now academia.

Sociology emerged as a discipline in the 18th century, at about the same time that people in British and French asylums began to be engaged in the occupations of farm work, housekeeping, and crafts. In enabling such outcasts to heal themselves and to discover their worth in society, occupation workers likely drew on growing medical knowledge of illness and new psychological insights on human development and motivation, as well as on knowledge emerging from sociology on occupation, deviance, mental illness, class, and society.

The professionalisation of occupational work as occupational therapy in the 20th century made the medical and psychological foundations of occupational therapy explicit. Occupational therapy education has stressed the importance of knowing anatomy, physiology, pathology, psychology, and medical conditions for working with individuals in medical settings. Unfortunately, this emphasis left the sociological foundations of occupational therapy as implicit, taken-for-granted, common knowledge. Fortunately, researchers inside and outside occupational therapy are retrieving and advancing the social knowledge which can inform occupational therapists about this profession and our interests in ageing, disability, culture, and more.

The editors have made a major contribution by gathering the ideas of 18 authors into a text which makes sociology explicit as a foundation for occupational therapy practice. Derek Jones introduces sociology and occupational therapy by acknowledging that these two fields share the dilemma of articulating what appears to be common knowledge and common sense. Jones then argues that sociology is an 'essential element of reflective practice' for occupational therapists who focus on the dialectical process of persons engaging in daily life in an environment. His argument is supported by six important reasons for occupational therapists to extend their use of sociology to both guide and understand practice.

As the chapters unfold, readers enter a world where sociology and occupational therapy are brought together. Early on in the book, we learn that one overriding reason for reading sociology is that social theories and research methods can advance knowledge about the quality and social contribution of occupational therapy. Asking 'what is sociology?', Derek Jones and Terry Hartery lead the reader on an introductory tour of sociology and 'sociological imagination'. We hear how sociological perspectives (structural consensus theory, structural conflict theory, interpretative theory, feminist theory, and postmodernism) offer diverse windows on occupational therapy.

The question, 'what is research?' is posed by Kenneth Jones & Margaret Nicol who link sociological perspectives with ideas for occupational therapists to use positivist and antipositivist research, particularly ethnography, phenomenology, ethnomethodology, and social constructionism.

Convinced that sociology and social research methods are indeed a foundation for occupational therapy, I was drawn to chapters on the sociology of occupation, work and leisure; topics which are central to occupational therapy's concern with occupation in daily life. Asking 'what is work', Chris Yuill and Ian McMillan highlight the social construction of work, particularly in relation to culture and gender, and as a source not only of income, but also of structure, social status, and social relationships. Then Louise Thibodaux and Anita Bundy offer an evocative image of a fly-fisherman wading into a stream to illustrate the social idea that leisure is time for relaxation, pursuit of cultural meaning in a habitual weekend pattern, and status and social relationships which create a particular interior attitude of leisure in the fisherman. I was also drawn to the discussions on class, gender, and race, first summarised, then related to occupational therapy clients. For instance, occupation (defined as work) is often used as an indicator of class, as in the British Registrar-General's classification of occupations; gender and race are key characteristics which strongly determine what occupations are open to clients.

Turning a sociological lens on ourselves as well as our clients, Terry Hartery and Thomas Gahagan prompt reflection on the social stratification of class, and the middle class position of the occupation of occupational therapy. Doreen MacWhannell and Sheena Blair further illuminate occupational therapy's social position as a profession. Isabel Dyck's discussion of multiculturalism reminds us that 'time may be a constraint in practice, but a narrative approach in problem-solving with clients is more conducive to working within the complexities of cultural difference'. Furthermore, as an occupational therapist, I found invaluable the chapters on health and illness, deviance, and normalisation.

Derek and Kenneth Jones contrast the biomedical model of health and illness with lay perspectives, particularly the World Health Organisation's definition of health as 'a positive state of physical, psychological, and social well being' (Taylor & Field 1993), which they remind us is far more compatible than the biomedical model with occupational therapy's broad view of health. Derek Jones pushes us further to consider how medical and psychological theories of deviance locate notions of difference in the individual, whereas, social theories offer social explanations of difference. Kirsten Stalker and Chris Jones expand on ideas of deviance by reviewing theories of normalisation which have fostered individualised, biomedical models of disability, in contrast to critical, social models of disability. And what about the sociological foundations of occupational therapy's ideas about roles, the family, and organisation embedded in the American Model of Human Occupation, championed by Gary Kielhofner, and the Australian Model of Occupational Role Performance, articulated by Hillman and Chapparo? Sheena Blair (on role), Chris Ravetz (on family), and Carol Lennie and Linda Renton (on organisations) raise important issues of power and the cultural organisation of communities as elements of the social context which should prompt occupational therapists to re-visit our ideas about roles, family, and organisations.

Not to be forgotten is the sociology of professions: here are important points of analysis and critique for the future of occupational therapy. Kenneth Jones and Averil Stewart remind us that functionalist approaches define the traits of professions, whereas conflict and action approaches analyse professional power and autonomy. They tantalise us to pursue sociology by introducing current ideas on women in professions, and the effects of managerialism and the disability movement on occupational therapy.

Sociology and occupational therapy has been well edited to achieve a clear, accessible style of writing. Nevertheless, there is much to absorb in this book. For new readers to sociology, my advice to avoid being overwhelmed is to follow what I will call four editorial 'guideposts'.

Guidepost 1: authors explain topics in terms of some or all of the social theories emphasised in the book: functionalism, interactionism, Marxism, feminism, postmodernism;
Guidepost 2: there is a consistent thread of recognition of the contributions of qualitative as well as quantitative research;
Guidepost 3: every chapter presents a topic from sociological perspectives, followed by applications of this knowledge in occupational therapy;

Guidepost 4: learning activities are embedded in each chapter.

The learning activities increase the usefulness of Sociology and occupational therapy because they prompt a synthesis of knowledge, critical reflection on issues, and self-reflection. For instance, how would you answer Activity 2.3, 'To which of the perspectives described here do you find yourself drawn, and why?', Activity 10.3 'What does being healthy mean to you? Do you think that you are healthy?', or Activity 13.8, 'Find out what schemes exist in your area to help disabled people or people with mental health problems to gain employment'.

By the end of this book, as the editors wish, occupational therapists will appreciate the importance of studying sociology, and sociologists will have illustrations from a health profession, occupational therapy, which is relatively unknown on the sociological map.

REFERENCES

Taylor S, Field D 1993 Sociology of Health & Health Care. Blackwell Scientific, Oxford

Halifax, Nova Scotia, Canada, 1998   Elizabeth Townsend

1

Introduction

D. Jones

THE NEED FOR THIS BOOK

Despite the fact that there seem to be many text-books on sociology, there is a need for a book specifically relating this area to that of occupational therapy. First, many books aimed at the health professions tend to draw most of their illustrations from nursing. Second, there are areas of particular interest to occupational therapists, such as work and leisure, that tend not to appear in medical sociology texts.

Another factor taken in consideration in producing this book is that many readers will have had no previous contact with sociology or any of the other so-called social sciences. Indeed, you may be wondering why you are studying this subject at all. The need to learn anatomy and physiology may appear to be obvious, if arduous. Psychology, too, might seem to have a clear claim to its place in the curriculum. Sociology, on the other hand, may seem to be of limited use in helping you to help your clients, particularly if the person teaching you is unable to relate the material directly to the practice of occupational therapy. This book intends to prove that sociology is not only an interesting subject, but also an essential element of reflective practice.

COMMON PROFESSIONAL STRUGGLES

In some respects sociologists and occupational therapists have much in common. Undergraduates in both disciplines often have difficulty

1

in defining their chosen field; tutors in both areas will be familiar with the cry from students, 'But what *is* sociology/occupational therapy?' The truth of the matter is, for this author at least, that both occupational therapy and sociology deal with in essence deceptively simple concerns. The former is about helping people to attain the life they would like, the latter deals with why our day-to-day lives take the form they do. Achieving one requires an understanding of the other.

Another shared experience of occupational therapists and sociologists is hearing the query 'But isn't what you do just common sense?' In some ways, this is true but only if we appreciate that common sense is not always conscious sense. That is to say, our knowledge of the world is often buried deep inside us, and it is only by careful analysis that it can be brought to mind. Take activity analysis as an example. Show someone a breakdown of the activity of pouring a glass of wine and they may be unimpressed; ask them to undertake a similar analysis and it is unlikely that they will find the task to be easy. Similarly, we all know what a family is – or do we? Would everyone consider a gay couple with children to be a family? Occupational therapy and sociology are often about getting beneath the surface of things, whether that is investigating why a person is developing a bad back at work or why people in manual jobs tend to suffer more ill-health.

HOW TO USE THIS BOOK

Each chapter in this book has two elements. In general, the first part of each chapter will introduce you to the basic sociological concepts and theories relating to that topic. There will inevitably be some omissions: a book of this size cannot hope to introduce you to everything sociologists have had to say on a particular topic. We have focused on what we consider to be key areas for you to understand and have attempted to introduce some of the sociological terminology. Note that some people will disparagingly refer to this terminology as 'jargon' yet be quite happy to accept the 'jargon' of anatomy: flexion, extension, etc. Terminology is used within a discipline to help

clear communication and understanding of complex concepts. It is just as important that you use this language correctly in sociology as in anatomy.

The second element of each chapter is written by an occupational therapist, who will attempt to tell you why and how the information contained in the first part is of relevance to them. They will tell you how they integrate this knowledge and how it informs their practice (hence the title of the book). They may not make reference to all the material contained in the first part as their contribution is very much a personal view. You may also very well be able to make some links that are not highlighted.

The book is constructed so that you can dip into any of the chapters in any order, but we would recommend that you read Chapter 2, 'Welcome to sociology', first. There will inevitably be some overlap between chapters; in some ways the division of topics into separate chapters is artificial in the same way as it is artificial to categorize fieldwork practice into physical or psychiatric services. Just as there may be mental health issues for someone with a physical impairment, so there will be gender issues to do with work, and class issues to do with leisure. We hope, however, that any overlap between chapters will take the form of reinforcement of knowledge rather than simple repetition. Additionally, the way in which one author explains a concept may make more sense to you than the approach of another.

Throughout the book, there are activities and questions to enable you to reflect on the material presented. We use this format not only to help you engage with the material, but also to help you think about the issues in relation to your own cultural setting.

About the chapters

In order to give you a taste of what to expect, there follows a brief outline of some of the key topics in each chapter.

Chapter 2 deals with the nature of sociology and its relationship to the other social sciences, introducing some of the main approaches within sociology and how they view society. This chapter provides much background information that will help in understanding some of the material contained in later chapters. It explains, for example, what is meant by a functionalist approach and how this differs from an inter-pretavist view of society. The second part of Chapter 2 looks at the influence of sociology on occupational therapy, considering how different sociological perspectives can be used to analyse the nature of therapeutic interventions.

The topic of methodology is covered in Chapter 3, which introduces some of the method-ological approaches used within sociology and how occupational therapists have utilized these research strategies. The chapter also considers that while sociologists have been critical of quan-titative methods, such approaches are still of value to occupational therapists. This chapter highlights the current emphasis on triangulation: the use of a variety of methodological approaches to study a particular topic.

In Chapter 4 you will learn how sociologists have theorized about the way in which members of a society can be identified as belonging to different stratified groups. In particular, it deals with the notion of social class and how mem-bership of a particular class can have a dramatic effect on a person's life – and death. The occupa-tional therapy element of the chapter looks at the implications of belonging to a particular class for occupational therapists. It also looks at how we have to broaden our notion of intervention if we accept that social conditions have an influence on people's health.

In looking at role, Chapter 5 deals with a con-cept with which occupational therapists are very familiar, although they do not necessarily appre-ciate its sociological sophistication. This often leads to a poor understanding of the concept and such terms as 'sick role'. The chapter looks at the different sociological perspectives on role and concepts such as role-set and role conflict. The place of role in the writing of an international range of occupational therapy theoreticians, such as Kielhofner from the USA and Hillman & Chapparo from Australia, is highlighted.

Issues of sex and gender have particular resonance for a profession that is largely female.

Like class, issues of gender appear in many of the chapters, but in Chapter 6, the difference between sex and gender is highlighted and issues of sex-role stereotyping are explored. The chapter also looks at the feminist critique of sociology. In relation to occupational therapy, the development of the profession as 'women's work' is examined, and issues of sex-role stereo-typing in clinical practice are addressed. You will also be introduced to what has become known as the 'feminine principle' in occupational therapy.

Chapter 7 highlights the fact that most Western occupational therapists practise in multicultural societies. It deals with an important topic that is only just beginning to receive the space in professional journals that it deserves. Issues such as the notion of culture, ethnicity and race are covered. Implications for therapists working in a multicultural setting are explored, and the notion of 'cultural safety' in fieldwork practice will be introduced.

In focusing on the family, we are once again confronted with the problem of definition, and Chapter 8 explores different forms of family structure. Different perspectives on the value of the family are given, and in particular, issues concerning the family and health will be debated. This element is of particular relevance to occupa-tional therapists given the increasing importance of the family in relation to community-based care.

Chapter 9 looks at the value-laden topic of deviance. The way in which sociologists have attempted to explain behaviour to which others respond negatively is explored and contrasted with psychological and biological explanations of 'deviant behaviour'. The second element of the chapter looks at the influence of labelling theory, in particular issues of direct relevance to occupational therapists in terms of the language they use and the nature of services to people with learning difficulties.

Some of the main issues and perspectives concerned with the sociology of health and ill-ness are introduced in Chapter 10. The develop-ment of our ideas about health and the way in which we think about our bodies is outlined. In this chapter, the reader is introduced to the issue of power and control in the professional–

client relationship. This chapter highlights why it is important for occupational therapists to be aware of their own, and their clients', understanding of health and illness. Chronic pain features in the lives of many people with whom occupational therapists will find themselves working. Thus the impact of chronic pain on self-identity is used to explore some implications for intervention that are applicable to chronic illnesses in general.

Chapter 11 highlights the way in which sociologists have looked at organizations, an important topic as all occupational therapists will come into contact with organizations, whether as employees or in acting on their clients' behalf. It outlines the different ways in which theorists have defined organizations as well as broader issues concerned with power, bureaucracy and society. In relation to occupational therapy, the problems associated with working within an organization are explored, as is the changing nature of health- and social care organizations.

Chapter 12 deals with a topic of crucial importance to any self-reflecting student or practitioner: the very nature of professions and professionals. This chapter looks at issues such as which occupations can be defined as professions and whether professionals, particularly medical professionals, act in their clients' or their own interests. In relation to occupational therapy, you will be encouraged to decide whether your chosen career is designated a profession in sociological terms. You will also read about the challenge to the power of professionals coming from disabled people.

Occupational therapists have long had an interest in work, and Chapter 13 examines some of the difficulties in defining work and considers some of the positive and negative aspects of this part of life, which carries so much importance. Key concepts such as the division of labour, alienation and the Protestant work ethic are discussed. The second element of this chapter looks at the way in which sociological knowledge can inform vocational rehabilitation. There is a focus on understanding the meaning of work for one's clients and the implications of the existence of high rates of long-term unemployment.

Chapter 14 looks at leisure and has a natural affinity with Chapter 13, particularly in relation to the problem of definition. The different ways in which leisure has been conceptualized – as a kind of time, as a freely chosen activity and as a state of mind – are explored, and classical perspectives are outlined. Within occupational therapy, the complex nature of leisure is sometimes not made explicit. In this chapter, the importance for therapists of seeing leisure in multidimensional terms is highlighted, particular attention being paid to issues concerning assessment and intervention.

The final chapter, 'Normalization and critical disability theory', is unique in that it deals with an area some would say has traditionally been poorly served by sociologists. This chapter deals with the work being produced by disabled academics and activists that challenges traditional notions of disability. In particular, the World Health Organisation's classification of impairment, disease and handicap is examined and compared with a social model of disability. The second part of the chapter outlines how occupational therapy practice has reflected and could, if not must, change in response to changing ideas of disability.

AN INTERNATIONAL PERSPECTIVE

Where possible, chapter authors have tried to draw on an international range of literature, which has inevitably tended to be restricted to works published in the English language which have a British/North American orientation. Nevertheless, we believe that many issues will strike a chord regardless of country. Cultural differences are very important and will affect the practice of occupational therapy between countries. However, it is also true that there are many similar issues for therapists working in any industrialized capitalist society at the end of the twentieth century.

The editors would like to develop the international perspective of the book and would welcome comments, literature recommendations or illustrations of the relevance of sociology from therapists world wide. This will enable us to give the book more international validity in any future editions.

2

What is sociology?

T. Hartery   D. Jones

Most schools of occupational therapy now include sociology somewhere in their curriculum, reflecting the importance of the subject. This chapter covers what sociology is and why it is important for occupational therapy students to know something about it. Readers will be introduced to what it is about the way in which sociologists study the world that distinguishes sociology from other social sciences, and to the ways in which different sociologists have studied society. How the influence of sociology can be seen in the work of occupational therapists will also be investigated. Later chapters will look in more detail at the specific contribution of the discipline to areas of particular interest to therapists.

HOW SOCIOLOGY DEVELOPED

Sociology began to develop in France around the time of the French Revolution as Auguste Comte (1798–1857), sometimes called the father of sociology, sought to understand the effects of the Revolution on French society. Since Comte, sociologists have continued to study societies in order to try to understand how they work and how and why they are changing. However, sociology does not concern itself with all human societies: it is usually taken to be the study of Western industrial societies. This means that sociology concentrates on trying to understand societies such as Britain, North America, Norway and Germany. These societies have undergone the process known as industrialization and, as a result, have developed particular features, for example, class systems, science and technology, the predominance of urban living, welfare states, and so on. All of this means that sociology is different from other related subjects such as:

- anthropology
- psychology
- social psychology.

Anthropology

Anthropology is usually regarded as the study of non-industrial, often peasant or tribal societies that are organized very differently from societies in the West. Such societies are often based upon the extended family or the clan, are not part of a money economy and live by very different rules and values from those of the West.

Psychology

Coon (1994) defines psychology as 'the scientific study of human and animal behaviour'. However, looking at the range of topics studied – memory, stress, perception, sexuality and personality to name but a few – it is clear that psychology studies not just behaviour, but also the mental processes and states of mind that underlie and influence such behaviour. What is also apparent is that psychology concentrates on individuals, the inner processes that are responsible for their functioning and why, as individuals, they differ from one another. As a generalization, it can be said that psychologists, unlike sociologists or social psychologists, are less interested in the workings of society or the impact of groups on individuals than they are in the study of individuals themselves. This can be illustrated by the fact that, while sociologists may be interested in the sources of stress in society, psychologists will concern themselves with the ways in which individuals cope with stress, in order to suggest better ways of dealing with it.

Social psychology

Social psychology is defined as 'the study of how individuals are influenced by other people – their social environment' (Brewer & Crano 1994). As such, social psychology concentrates on how individuals relate to one another in social groups and how these groups in turn affect individuals. Areas of concern for social psychologists include the study of attitudes and social perception, affiliation and attraction, conformity, consensus and intergroup relations.

It is often difficult to tell where sociology ends and psychology, more particularly social psychology, begins. To a large extent, this is an unimportant question, but, broadly speaking, we can say that sociology is more concerned with identifying the influence of society, as a whole, on people in general rather than with the specific influences on Joe Bloggs in particular. It is more interested in what we have in common than in the ways in which we are different from each other.

SOCIAL PATTERNING – THE BASIS OF SOCIOLOGY

The development of the social sciences, each with its own distinctive subject matter, shows that a range of explanations are required to explain human behaviour in all its complexity. Each subject area makes valid contributions to this study by explaining certain aspects of behaviour with which the others, with their different focus, are less well equipped to deal. Psychologists, for example, with their concentration on the individual, are better equipped to explain why some people in a particular social situation respond to that situation differently from others.

It has to be recognized, however, that individuals in society do not usually 'do their own thing'. It is clear that, in daily life, people tend to act in the same way again and again in particular social settings, so what is seen is:

not chaos and confusion but a reasonable approximation of order: motorists [in Britain] drive on the left-hand side of the road, not on the right; shoppers offer coins and banknotes, cheques and cheque cards in exchange for goods and services, not goats and chickens or nothing at all; love-making takes place indoors in bedrooms, not outside on the pavement. (Bilton et al 1987)

This means that human social behaviour exhibits patterns or regularities and is therefore predictable. It also means that these behaviours can be explained with reference to social forces. The existence of regularities in social behaviour caused or influenced by social forces is the basis of sociology and the sociological perspective (Activity 2.1).

Activity 2.1

What regularities in social behaviour can you identify?

INVESTIGATING SOCIETY AT DIFFERENT LEVELS

The fact that social behaviour exhibits regularities that persist over time allows sociologists to study and make statements about the types of behaviour typically found in a society and to explain why it exists. In order to illustrate the areas of interest for sociologists, it can be said that sociology studies society on three different levels (Inkeles 1964):

1. society as a whole
2. social institutions
3. social relationships.

Society as a whole

This level of analysis is sometimes called the macro level. Here, sociologists ask such questions as 'What sort of society is it (capitalist, communist or early industrial?)', 'Through what stages of development has it passed?', 'What are the factors that cause it to change?', 'How does it manage problems?' and 'How does it survive over time?' The basic perspective at this level is to see society as being made up of a number of interrelated institutions such as the family and education.

Social institutions

Institutions such as the family, church, school and political parties have important consequences for society and can therefore be studied in their own right rather than just as part of the big picture. At the intermediate, or meso, level, instead of asking such questions as 'How does this society work?', the questions are 'How does this particular institution work?', 'How did it come into being?', 'What are its effects?' and 'How is it changing?' Several chapters in the book deal with issues at this level.

Social relationships

Social institutions are in turn made up of sets of social relationships, for example the relationship between parents and children in the family or teachers and pupils in a school. Some of the most interesting sociological studies have been carried out at this micro level. Goffman (1969), for one, argues that we engage all the time in 'impression management', that is, through speech, behaviour and dress, we are trying to convey favourable impressions of ourselves to others because we stand to lose and gain from our relationships with them. This in turn raises interesting questions about whether people are ever really natural or spontaneous, or whether they consciously plan out performances to impress people. A good example of impression management is when people go for interview: they dress smartly and talk and act in ways that maximize their chances of success. Whilst such behaviour is understandable and sensible, it does illustrate the ways in which our actions are consciously managed in our relations with others.

If sociology is the study of society at different levels, the next question is 'How is this done?' This is the province of sociological methodology (see Chapter 3), but underlying any attempt to study society is the need to develop what C. Wright Mills calls 'the sociological imagination'.

SOCIOLOGICAL IMAGINATION

This refers to 'The quality of mind essential to grasp the interplay of man and society, of biography and history, of self and world' (Mills 1959). According to Mills, individuals live in particular types of society with particular histories: these individuals are formed by these societies and, in turn through their behaviour, help to recreate them through the millions of acts that they perform in their daily lives. From this perspective, therefore, to talk about a separation between the society and the individual is artificial since each affects the other. It means that people can only understand themselves as individuals if they grasp this fact for, as Mills says, 'the individual can understand his experience and gauge his own fate only by locating himself within his period, ... he can know his own chances of life only by becoming aware of those of all individuals in his circumstances'.

In essence, then, sociological imagination means the ability to detach oneself from familiar routines and look at them anew in order to understand the interplay between society and the individual. To facilitate this, it is necessary to develop a cross-cultural and historical perspective through the study of subjects such as anthropology, history and economics.

These are very important ideas because people tend to see the world from the perspective of their own narrow upbringing and experience. What Mills is saying is that it is necessary to examine our limited experience, to see how it differs from the experience of others, both in our own society as well as in societies very different from our own, in order to learn more about why we do things as we do (developing a cross-cultural and historical perspective here is crucial in allowing this to be done). It also means becoming aware of the ways in which people's lives are affected and constrained by the society in which they live. Developing the sociological imagination thus means stopping explaining things purely in individualistic terms and instead looking to the social forces (culture, class, group pressure, position and income) that influence or constrain people to act in particular ways.

One example of using the sociological imagination comes from education. The most common explanation for educational success is that it results from individual ability. People holding this belief think that those who achieve high educational qualifications do so because they are the most intelligent in society. Using the sociological imagination, however, a number of surprising things emerge.

To begin with, there is a wealth of evidence showing that upper- and middle-class children are much more likely to go on to higher education than are working-class children. Intelligence is not the crucial factor here because studies show that, when comparing middle-class and working-class children with the same intelligence, the middle-class children are still more likely to go on to higher education. The reason for these educational differences seems instead to lie with the very different backgrounds of these children and the social forces that influence their lives (in particular their parents' attitudes to education, the level of family resources and the way in which schools treat children from different class backgrounds). The educational experience of working-class children is thus very different from that of other children because their position in society and that of their parents opens them up to social and economic influences different from those of other children. Appreciating this may help to understand the jobs that they do or do not get, their relatively limited chances in life and why their attitudes may be different from those of more educated groups. A similar analysis can be made of educational differences between men and women, and between white children and those from ethnic minorities.

COMPETING EXPLANATIONS OF SOCIAL BEHAVIOUR

Using the sociological imagination may therefore lead to seeing and understanding things in ways quite different from before. In particular, it cautions against explaining behaviour in purely individualistic terms. Bilton et al (1987) illustrate and expand upon this point with their distinction between sociological, naturalistic and individualistic explanations of behaviour.

NATURALISTIC EXPLANATIONS

While sociological explanations, as we have seen,

emphasize the influence of social factors on behaviour, naturalistic or biological explanations argue that, like other animals, human beings are biologically programmed by nature to behave in certain ways (sociobiologists such as Desmond Morris being one group who use this type of explanation). Naturalistic explanations state, for example, that it is natural for men and women to fall in love, marry and have children. Part of the reason why this is said to be so is that women have a maternal instinct that needs to be satisfied through childbearing. The same biological argument is advanced to explain why it is natural for men to be workers (they are genetically programmed to be more aggressive and competitive) and for women to be housewives and mothers (because they are naturally more submissive and caring).

Bilton et al (1987) argue that such naturalistic explanations should be rejected because they present an entirely distorted picture of social reality, which ignores the role of social factors in affecting what is considered to be 'human nature'. Anthropological evidence shows that 'human nature' varies from society to society (illustrating the value of the cross-cultural perspective to sociology) and is dependent on a range of social, economic and political factors operating in a particular society. In the case of women being considered as 'naturally' housewives and mothers, Oakley (1974), shows that the role of housewife did not exist before the Industrial Revolution (illustrating the value of an historical perspective). Women only became established in the housewife role once industrialization was under way, mainly because of the effects of various factory acts that prohibited the employment of children and through the efforts of male-dominated trade unions to secure jobs for men. As this example shows, women's roles are more the product of social expectations than any maternal or other instinct.

The other objection to naturalistic explanations is that they justify the *status quo*. If something exists because it is 'natural', then, by definition, it cannot easily be changed. Sociologists worry that such explanations are often used to maintain people in unequal positions because it is to the benefit of more privileged groups. It could be argued, for example, that the growing argument in the USA that crime has a genetic cause is one example of a naturalistic explanation being used by powerful and wealthy groups to ignore the sociological argument that crime has a lot to do with poverty and unemployment. This is because the recognition of such a viewpoint could potentially affect their position if, as a result, they were required to redistribute some of their wealth to the poor.

INDIVIDUALISTIC EXPLANATIONS

Individualistic explanations are ones that explain behaviour in terms of the psychological make-up of individuals. For example, criminals are people who lack any idea of right or wrong, the unemployed are lazy and feckless, and successful people are more clever and more hard-working than less successful people. Individualistic explanations are discounted by sociologists on the grounds that, by ignoring the role of social factors and explaining behaviour purely in terms of the individuals involved, they give an inadequate explanation of what occurs. It may be true that, in a particular situation, individual factors are involved, but they cannot by themselves account for the totality observed. As an illustration, much of the media reporting of the poll tax demonstrations in Britain in the late 1980s blamed agitators for what occurred. While there may have been some truth to this such an account cannot explain why so many people turned up for these events and allowed themselves to led in particular ways. A more reasonable explanation for the demonstrations would be the sociological one that large numbers of people came to gather in groups because they felt the poll tax to be unjust and wished to make the government aware of how they felt. Individualistic explanations, especially when concerned with issues of poverty or health,

Activity 2.2
Make a note of what you understand by the terms 'sociological', 'naturalistic' and 'individualistic'.

are sometimes known as 'victim blaming' because they blame individuals for their own misfortunes instead of looking for the causes in the wider society.

SOCIOLOGY AND COMMON SENSE

Naturalistic and individualistic explanations abound and often comprise the bulk of what is called 'common sense' in a society. Sociologists have two main objections to common-sense explanations: first, they ignore the role of social factors in behaviour, and second, they are untested. The first objection has been dealt with above; the second must await the chapter on methodology and the place of sociology as a social science before it is clarified. Hopefully, however, enough has already been written to explain why sociologists would not accept the statement that sociology is just common sense.

SOCIOLOGICAL PERSPECTIVES

One thing that quickly becomes clear to people studying sociology for the first time is that sociology does not have one unified view of society but instead comprises a number of views or perspectives. A perspective is a point of view, a particular way of looking at and explaining the world. The same event may appear entirely different in meaning to two people who view it from different perspectives (Berry 1976).

Just as different individuals and groups may hold different perspectives (think of the differences between Conservative and Labour politicians in Britain on such issues as rail privatization, homelessness and Europe, or the traditional disagreement on budget deficits between the Republicans and the Democrats in the USA), so sociologists have not been in agreement about the way in which society works or the reasons for particular behaviours within society. The result has been the development of a number of perspectives or schools of thought, which, although they often contain mutually incompatible assumptions, nevertheless provide the basis

for an 'organized controversy' over key social issues. Thus, while different perspectives dealing with, for example, the macro level of society as a whole will explain the existence and persistence of society differently, they still agree that certain things are worth studying and certain things are not (for example questions of consensus and conflict, rather than ego states and dream analysis).

The existence of different perspectives is held to be desirable because it provides a check to complacently held assumptions about social life emanating from society itself, leads to the possibility of the critical scrutiny of research reports to uncover narrow or fallacious thinking and helps to clarify the proper concerns of the discipline (Lee & Newby 1983).

Five distinct types of sociological perspective will be dealt with here to illustrate how sociologists have thought about society and the various kinds of social forces that affect human behaviour. In addition to laying the foundations for sociological understanding, this will also provide an outline for understanding the content of other chapters in the book.

STRUCTURAL CONSENSUS THEORY

Structural consensus theory takes as its starting point the argument that each society has a culture consisting of a set of rules and values that structure or channel the behaviour of its members in particular ways. This culture exists prior to the birth of new members of society so has to be learned by them through the process known as socialization. Through socialization, new members of society internalize the culture and thus act in conformity with its norms and values. In addition, socialization produces an agreement or consensus between people on what is appropriate behaviour. Through socialization, therefore, cultural rules structure behaviour, guarantee a consensus about expected behaviour and thereby ensure social order (Jones 1993).

Functionalism is the best-known development of structural consensus theory. It became the dominant social theory in the 1940s and 50s, although it has since lost ground. Functionalism is associated with several of the 'big names' in sociology (Durkheim, Parsons and Merton), each of whom added their own elaborations to the theory. Some of the key elements of functionalism are shown in Box 2.1.

Box 2.1 Key elements of functionalism

- Each society has certain social needs or functional prerequisites that must be met if the society is to survive. These prerequisites include the need to reproduce new generations, provide food and clothing, control conflict and maintain social order and social solidarity

- Societies meet these social needs by developing structures or institutions (conceived of as structures of rules or social roles) that carry out functions. The function of any activity or structure is the part it plays in maintaining the society. Thus, for example, every society develops some form of family to reproduce and socialize new generations

- Society is viewed as a whole made up of interrelated and interdependent parts. Thus institutions such as the family, education and the economy carry out functions that, together, help society to survive

- The whole society is held together by a value consensus. Each society has a culture consisting of core norms and values. People learn the norms through socialization and follow them because they believe them to be morally correct. The result of such rule-following is social order and stability

---

A number of important implications follow from functionalism. Since institutions exist to help society survive, it follows that they are to be seen as beneficial for society and the individual. They should therefore be supported rather than criticized or challenged. Some sociologists would argue from this that functionalism works to support the *status quo*. Since a value consensus prevails, this implies that harmony and cooperation are the dominant social processes. From this perspective, conflict is aberrant and to be eradicated rather than being seen as a positive force for change in society. The fact that functionalism stresses the role of culture or social rules in determining behaviour denies the spontaneity and non-conformity seen in society as well as emphasizing 'cultural' explanations over other types, for example materialist explanations.

STRUCTURAL CONFLICT THEORY

These theories agree that society determines behaviour by structuring or constraining it but emphasize different factors, namely the distribution of advantage and disadvantage. Thus people are not only constrained by the norms and values that they have learnt via socialization, but also by their position in the structure of inequality in society (Jones 1993). Following this argument, for example, poor people in a class society may find it more difficult to maintain their health compared with the more affluent because they cannot afford a healthy diet.

Marxism is an example of structural conflict theory. Marx (1818–83) argued that the primary division in capitalist society is between an owning class (the bourgeoisie or capitalists), which owns the means of production (factories, etc.), and the workers (proletariat), who do not, thus having to sell their labour for wages to the owners. The ownership of the means of production allows the capitalists to exploit the workers, who, as a result, live lives characterized by poverty, misery and oppression. Since the interests of the owners are opposed to those of the workers, Marxism sees conflict between the two groups as a normal feature of capitalist society and likewise explains the workers' behaviour and health status as a result of their position in a system of material advantage and disadvantage. Marxism is therefore offering a materialist rather than cultural explanation. Unlike functionalism, which stresses the impact of norms and values on behaviour, Marxism argues that behaviour is affected by material factors such as poverty and exploitation. This distinction becomes important when considering the Black Report in Chapter 4.

INTERPRETATIVE THEORY

Within sociology, there are a group of theories that are quite different from structuralist theories. These theories may also sometimes be called action or interactionist theories. While this perspective is often associated with more modern sociologists such as Goffman, it has its roots in the work of Max Weber (1864–1920) and Georg Simmel (1858–1918).

Instead of explaining behaviour from the point of view of how society structures behaviour (as is the case with the structural consensus and structural conflict theories), this perspective focuses on the way in which the interaction between individuals involves processes of interpretation that lead them to assign meaning to each other's behaviour before deciding how to act. Since interpretative theory concerns itself with small-scale interactions between individuals, it is known as microtheory, in contrast with structural theories that consider society as a whole and are therefore known as macrotheories. With interpretative theory, the order that is seen in social life occurs not through the blind following of social norms or because people are constrained by inequality, but because individuals have the ability to work out (interpret) what is going on around them and then choose how to act in the light of this interpretation.

Symbolic interactionism is an example of interpretative theory. According to Blumer (1962), the essence of symbolic interactionism is that people act on the basis of meanings they attach to objects and events rather than by simply reacting to social forces such as culture. The notion of meaning refers to an interpretation of the significance of a situation, act, idea or object with reference to how one should respond (Open University 1975) Before individuals can act in a situation, they have to assign a meaning to it or, to use W. I. Thomas' phrase, to define their situation. This means they have to work out mentally what the situation means to them on the basis of their interpretation of the various signs and cues that are present. Seeing someone lying on the ground, for example, can be interpreted in a number of ways: is the person dead, injured, drunk and so on? The meaning people assign to the situation will influence how they act – call for an ambulance or the police, or walk away in disgust.

Meanings often emerge during interaction rather than simply being there from the beginning This construction of meaning involves a process of negotiation and bargaining between participants that results in meanings being created, modified and changed. Thus, for example, when the police are called to a disturbance, they may begin by arresting those whom they believe to be troublemakers but later let them go after those arrested are able to convince the police that what happened was just high spirits.

This basic interactionist perspective has been applied in a number of ways, for example in labelling theory and the process of stigmatization (see Chapter 9), as well as in the analysis of everyday role situations (see Chapter 5). In relation to roles, interactionists argue that, like meanings generally, these provide vague guidelines for behaviour and are developed during interaction through processes of negotiation and bargaining. This means that roles are continually being recreated, as well as created and changed, by the activities of those involved in the situation. This leads to symbolic interactionists denying that culture determines behaviour; instead, culture itself is created and recreated by actors in interaction situations (see the section on cultural variation in Chapter 7). One example of such cultural change has been the changing role of women in Western industrial societies over the twentieth century. During this period, women have negotiated and bargained with men over what their respective roles should be, changing culture in significant ways in the process (Vander Zanden 1979).

FEMINIST THEORY

Feminist theories are concerned with the subordinate position of women in many societies and the explanation for these gender inequalities. Underlying this perspective is the realization that women are disadvantaged compared with men in areas such as household responsibilities, pay and status in work and in terms of career prospects. There is also the point that many other sociological theories, such as functionalism and Marxism, look at social life essentially from the perspective of men rather than women.

It is traditional to categorize feminism in terms of three main perspectives:

- liberal feminism
- radical feminism
- Marxist feminism.

However, as will be seen in Chapter 6, this categorization may not reflect more recent developments in feminist theory.

Liberal feminism

Liberal feminists believe that gender inequalities are basically the result of the socialization into gender roles that begins in early childhood, and discrimination at work, which prevents women receiving equal opportunities to men. The way to deal with this is through the promotion of antisexist attitudes and antidiscrimination legislation.

Radical feminism

Radical feminists argue that patriarchy – male domination – is the basic reason for women's subordination and inequality. From this perspective, all men exploit and oppress women. While this is accepted as basic by radical feminists, there is less agreement on why patriarchy exists.

Shulamith Firestone (1972), for example, believes that patriarchy and women's oppression is rooted in biology, in the fact that only women can bear children. Biology gave rise to the 'biological family' in which women, because of the long years involved in childrearing, became dependent on men, who were in turn able to dominate and oppress them. Firestone also believes that the biological family formed the basis of other forms of inequality, since men enjoyed their domination over women and wanted to extend it to domination over other men. Other radical feminists, for example Sherry Ortner (1974), see patriarchy as the result of a male control of ideas and culture, which allows women to be regarded and treated as inferior to men.

Radical feminists have different solutions to the problem of patriarchy. Some, like Firestone, believe that liberation will only come when it is possible to conceive and rear children outside the womb, thus reducing women's dependence on men and the biological family. Others believe that women should band together and organize their lives differently and separately from men.

Marxist feminism

These feminists regard the inferior position of women as the result of exploitation by the capitalist class. The expectation that women should be unpaid housewives and mothers, for example, is explained by the fact that capitalism benefits from having new generations of labour produced through their efforts at no cost to the employer. The way out of such situations is through revolution and the establishment of the Communist society.

POSTMODERNISM

Postmodernism is a perspective that has become popular in recent years; to understand it requires an awareness of the development of 'modern' society.

The origins of modern society lie with industrialization. Industrialization had a massive impact on the nature and functioning of medieval society, which was basically agricultural and characterized by a belief in tradition and religion. Industrialization gave rise to modern society, based on capitalistic methods of production (such as the market and the factory system), the development of the centralized state and the belief in reason as the basis for the progress or improvement of human life. The link between reason and progress was that it led to knowledge that could improve the human condition. This belief in reason as the basis for progress gave rise, among other things, to the sciences, which are an attempt to understand the world in order to control and improve it for the benefit of people. This applies to the social sciences as well as the natural sciences. Sociology, for example, grew out of Comte's attempt to understand, and therefore control, the consequences of the French Revolution. Later sociologists such as Marx wanted to understand capitalist society so that it could be changed for the better. Modernity, therefore, has an important cultural dimension that involves a challenge to 'tradition' in the name of rationality and a stress on the virtues of scientific and technical knowledge (Jones 1993).

Postmodernism is a recent development in

sociology arguing that we live in a postmodern society in which we are confronted with multiple realities that are ephemeral and constantly changing. From this perspective, nothing is permanent, nothing is certain, including the truth. The result is that social life is characterized by superficiality and uncertainty, fashion, trend and image, as a result, having come to mean more than substance and meaning (Jones 1993). Part of the reason for this state of affairs lies with the mass media, whose importance in modern life is that they construct reality for us via advertising, popular music and television soap operas. This reality is fragmentary, impermanent and inconsistent, and helps to create the sort of society in which what is believed today is different from what is believed tomorrow.

As a theory, then, one thing postmodernism does is to describe the experience of life for many in modern Western society as one in which the world is going mad, where change is too fast and nothing is reliable (Craib 1992). On another level, however, the theory has important implications for the search for truth and for sociology as a discipline. This follows because, as we have seen, part of its argument is that there is no one overall truth, no one overall reality. Instead, there are merely different and conflicting views of the world, which are all equally valid and equally ephemeral. Postmodernists therefore believe that there is no metanarrative, no grand theory of society. From this perspective, sociological theories such as Marxism and functionalism have no more claim to tell the truth than does any other source of knowledge.

Postmodernism and the end of sociology?

This chapter began by arguing that the sociological imagination involves the ability to look at the interrelationship between the individual and society and to offer sociological explanations that emphasize the role of social forces in affecting behaviour. Functionalism, Marxism and symbolic interactionism are all examples of attempts to offer such sociological explanations, with most sociologists using these or other

theoretical frameworks to analyse and understand the social world. Postmodernists believe that it is impossible to study society in this way. However, criticisms have started to emerge of postmodernism that it has overstated its case, and for this reason, many sociologists still believe that the search for a sociological understanding of society is a valid endeavour.

Activity 2.3

To which of the perspectives described here do find yourself drawn, and why?

WHY STUDY SOCIOLOGICAL PERSPECTIVES?

Given that sociologists are not agreed on how society works, it could be (and has been) argued that studying different perspectives is a waste of time. However, as stated earlier, from a sociologist's viewpoint, these perspectives form an organized controversy that helps to clarify the concerns of the discipline. From the point of view of the student coming to sociology, studying perspectives may make them aware, perhaps for the first time, of how complex social issues are and how sociologists see things very differently from non-sociologists. Craib (1992) makes a similar point when he argues that sociological perspectives provide us with the opportunity to become 'better citizens', more aware and with a deeper understanding of what is happening in the world. They do this not so much by providing answers to problems, but by allowing a better understanding of their complexity and difficulty. Realizing that social issues are complex and open to interpretation may help to prevent the search for simplistic, often naturalistic or individualistic, explanations and make people think before they act.

Sociological perspectives also make some propositions that are contrary to people's experiences and beliefs. Becoming aware of the discrepancies between theory and everyday thinking and behaviour can be the basis for individuals reassessing their lives and making appropriate changes. An illustration of this could be the way in which women are still brought up to see the roles of housewife and mother as primary in modern society. Marxism explains this in terms of the needs of capitalism for new generations of workers at the lowest cost. Women play an important part in this process, taking the main (unpaid) responsibility for child-rearing and housework even when holding down a job themselves. Feminism raises a similar argument, except that it is men rather than capitalism who are responsible. Looking at the issue in this sociological way may lead some women to believe that their roles are not biologically determined but socially constructed to meet the needs of certain groups.

Sociological perspectives can thus give us tools for looking at the world. We can use these tools both within occupational therapy and in reflecting on the profession itself.

SOCIOLOGY AND OCCUPATIONAL THERAPY

We may discern within the writings of some famous sociologists an affinity with the philosophy of occupational therapy. Georg Simmel (whose writings were, many years later, to influence the symbolic interactionists) noted, 'Experience seems to show that inner wholeness is created essentially in interaction with a complete rounded task in life' (quoted in Lawrence 1976, p. 202). This statement would seem to fit very well with the notion within occupational therapy of the importance of a balance of activities in daily life.

Hagedorn (1995), drawing our attention to the relatively recent place of sociology within the occupational therapy curriculum, suggests that sociological theory may have filtered into the profession without recognition or acknowledgement of the source. The rest of this chapter will explore salient points and connections of the different sociological perspectives in relation to occupational therapy, focusing in particular on:

- action theory

- functionalism
- Marxism
- feminism
- postmodernism.

OCCUPATIONAL THERAPY AND ACTION THEORY

We mentioned earlier in the chapter how Max Weber was one of the forerunners of an approach (action theory) that placed an emphasis on looking at the world from the perspective of the people involved in the situation being studied. Weber considered that sociology should not construct expert theories but should instead concern itself with seeking to understand the theories of actors themselves. The process by which this is done Weber called *verstehen* – putting oneself in the place of those whom we seek to understand and thereby appreciating the reasons for their actions (Bilton et al 1996). The affinity with occupational therapy's claim to client-centredness is clear.

The use of this perspective within occupational therapy can be seen in studies such as that undertaken by Jenkins et al (1994), looking at interactions between clients and graduates, diplomates, students and assistants. They identified the theoretical basis for their work by stating, 'The evidence from interactional analysis is that effective communication and therapy depend on an appreciation of the client's world.'

> **Activity 2.4**
>
> Have a look through the journal of your own professional association. Are there any articles that take an explicit interactionist perspective?

Further examination of Weber's views on industrialized society provide additional points for reflection, which may lead occupational therapists to consider both their own and their clients' positions. Weber saw modern life as being constrained and guided by rational action. By this, he means that people's behaviour is based on the calculation of the most efficient ways of achieving specific aims. Bureaucracy and 'marketization' are a reflection of this (Bilton et al 1987). The results of this process will be recognized by educators and clinicians, whom you may have heard express concern that students and clients are no longer felt to be individuals but 'consumers' or 'units' to be 'throughputted', their cost value having overriding importance. Bilton et al highlight Weber's concern about a world whose inhabitants live in a 'polar night of icy darkness' created by the neverending and ruthless rational pursuit of efficiency.

Activity 2.5

Do you feel that students and clients are becoming mere cogs in a machine, or does Weber have a romanticized view of life that ignores the benefits of efficiency and rational action? Discuss this issue with your tutors and clinicians.

OCCUPATIONAL THERAPY AND FUNCTIONALISM

The influence of a functionalist perspective within occupational therapy is largely implicit rather than explicit but can be seen in some of the literature relating to:

- roles
- Kielhofner's model of human occupation (MOHO).

Roles

Role theory is examined in more detail in Chapter 5, but it is worth highlighting some issues here. As we have seen, social roles are important within a functionalist perspective; people are thought to be socialized into various roles (parent, student, occupational therapist, etc.) that then, to a large extent, determine their behaviour. This approach is reflected in the statement of Kavanagh & Faves (1995), two occupational therapists working with homeless people, that 'Roles are a source of identity and are the frame work of everyday life.'

This view has been criticized both by sociologists from the interpretative perspective, who argue against the determinism inherent in this

view, and by occupational therapists such as Mocellin (1995), who believes the focus on roles to be stereotyping and that carrying out occupational roles, for example that of a housewife, may not always be therapeutic.

Activity 2.6

In what instances and why might the requirement to undertake a particular role not be considered therapeutic?

MOHO

The issue of roles is a key feature within MOHO, and it could be argued that this model reflects a functionalist perspective. Mocellin (1996) has highlighted the influence of MOHO on the profession; he notes the way in which the occupational therapy literature views the individual as an open system interacting with their environment. He highlights Kielhofner's view that the open system emphasizes function over structure. The concept of the open system is drawn from systems theory, which is also associated with the functionalist sociologist Talcott Parsons.

It would appear, then, that the MOHO is heavily influenced by a functionalist perspective. If this is the case, the model can also be subject to the same criticisms. While recognizing the acknowledgement within the MOHO and the writing of other American theorists, that people can influence their environments, the focus would seem to be on the individual adapting to the environment rather than vice versa. The, apparently, uncritical acceptance of the environment as it exists is also reflected in the definition of adaptation by one American postgraduate course as 'goodness of fit between people and their environments' (Yerxa 1993).

OCCUPATIONAL THERAPY AND MARXISM

We have already seen earlier in this chapter how structural conflict theorists, such as Marx, would challenge the assumption that the existing social system, or environment, is something to which we should adapt. The existing system is not necessarily the best, and some would argue that it should be changed.

In addition, Marx, like Simmel and Weber, was concerned with the way in which people exist in the world and how that existence is shaped. Marx had an optimistic view of humanity and saw the problems of society as resulting from particular forms of social organization rather than being natural. This is what is meant by people being constrained by circumstances, but it is important to remember the other element that stresses people's ability to act. Drawing on the earlier work of the philosopher Hegel, Marx identified that we create ourselves 'in a historical process, of which the motive force is human labour, or the practical activity of men living in society' (Bottomore & Rubel 1963, p. 18). In a statement that is surprisingly reminiscent of the idea of man being energized by the use of his hands (Reilly 1962), Marx also drew attention to the process of:

setting in motion arms and legs, head and hands, the natural forces of his body, in order to appropriate nature's productions in a form adapted to his own wants. (Marx 1867, quoted in Bottomore & Rubel 1963, p. 102)

Again drawing attention to the importance of varied activity in human life and the difficulty of achieving this in capitalist society, Marx noted how the division of labour traps us into particular lifestyles or activities:

He [sic] is a hunter, a fisherman, a shepherd, or a critical critic, and must remain so …; while in communist society where nobody has one exclusive sphere of activity but each can be accomplished in any branch he wishes, society regulates general production and thus makes it possible for one to do one thing to-day and another tomorrow … without ever becoming hunter, fisherman, shepherd or critic. (cited in Giddens 1971, p. 63)

The influence of Marx was explicitly acknowledged by Wilcox, who, speaking at a College of Occupational Therapists conference on health promotion in 1993, said that he was the first occupational scientist and noted the way in which he emphasized how labour is the collective creative activity of the people (Wilcox 1993).

OCCUPATIONAL THERAPY AND FEMINISM

Like Marx, most feminists would want to challenge the idea of individuals adapting to what could be seen as an oppressive system. Within occupational therapy, the value of a feminist perspective is being increasingly recognized. Articles in various journals have highlighted the affinity between some feminist perspectives and the philosophy of occupational therapy. For example, one whole issue of the *American Journal of Occupational Therapy* (vol. 46, no. 11) was given over to the topic in 1992. In other cases, the literature has highlighted the potential for stereotyping through the selection of activities dependent on the sex of the client, i.e. knitting for women and woodwork for men. This issue is explored further in Chapter 6.

OCCUPATIONAL THERAPY AND POSTMODERNISM

The impact of postmodernist perspectives on occupational therapy is only just beginning to be felt. 1996, for example, saw a conference organized by the British College of Occupational Therapy entitled 'The postmodern practitioner'. The same year, an article by Webber (1996), looking at the implications of postmodernism for occupational therapy, appeared in the *British Journal of Occupational Therapy*. It argued that this perspective challenges the claims to truth of scientific experts and suggested that outcomes data, measures of the effectiveness of therapy, should be acquired using qualitative methods. For Webber, the postmodernist practitioner is someone who adjusts his or her actions to meet the specific needs of clients based on the clients view of the world.

Webber's position is challenged by Hawes (1996) on the basis of postmodernism's inability to say anything for sure because of its emphasis on relativity. He argues that an overemphasis on the uniqueness of individuals fails to recognize wider objective structural constraints (poverty and the other inequalities inherent in capitalism), and that, for this reason, postmodernism is in fact antiholistic. Thus lack of income and the effects of this are facts that can be measured objectively. For Hawes, Marxism is the alternative because of the belief that, while human beings can have some control of their actions, they do not do so in circumstances of their own choosing.

CONCLUSION

We have seen how thinking sociologically means looking at the relationship between the individual and society and, in particular, at the ways in which social forces affect behaviour. Looking at things in this way can lead to new insights into social life that challenge conventional views, lead to disagreements with those who take a different line, and even unpopularity. On the other hand, sociological thinking can lead to more informed individuals and perhaps provide a basis for the reassessment of one's life. We have also seen how the mutual influence and affinity between sociology and occupational therapy can be discovered once we take the time and have the sociological knowledge to become aware of it. Welcome to sociology and the discovery of its relationship with occupational therapy.

REFERENCES

Berry D 1976 Central ideas in sociology. Constable, London

Bilton T, Bonnett K, Jones P, Skinner D, Stanworth M, Webster A 1987 Introductory sociology, 2nd edn. Macmillan, London

Blumer H 1962 Society as symbolic action. In: Rose A (ed.) Symbolic interactionism. Routledge & Kegan Paul, London

Bottomore T B, Rubel M 1963 Karl Marx: selected writings in sociology and social philosophy. Penguin, Harmondsworth

Brewer M, Crano W 1994 Social psychology. West Publishing Co., St Paul, Minneapolis

Coon D 1994 Essentials of psychology. West Publishing Co., St Paul, Minneapolis

Craib I 1992 Modern social theory. Harvester Wheatsheaf, Hemel Hempstead

Firestone S 1972 The dialectic of sex. Paladin, London

Giddens A 1971 Capitalism and modern social theory. Cambridge University Press, Cambridge

Goffman E 1969 The presentation of self in everyday life. Penguin, Harmondsworth

Hagedorn R 1995 Occupational therapy: perspectives and processes. Churchill Livingstone, Edinburgh

Hawes D 1996 Against postmodernism: a Marxist perspective. British Journal of Occupational Therapy 59 (3): 131–132

Inkeles A 1964 What is sociology? Prentice-Hall, Englewood Cliffs, NJ

Jenkins M, Mallet J, O'Neill C, McFadden M, Baird H 1994 Insights into 'practice' communication: an interactional approach. British Journal of Occupational Therapy 57(8): 297–302

Jones P 1993 Studying society: sociological theories and research practices. Collins Educational, London

Kavanagh J, Faves J 1995 Using the model of human occupation with homeless mentally ill clients. British Journal of Occupational Therapy 58(10): 419–422

Lawrence P 1976 Georg Simmel: sociologist and European. Nelson, Sunbury-on-Thames, Middx

Lee D, Newby H 1983 The problem of sociology: an introduction to the discipline. Hutchinson, London

Mills C W 1959 The sociological imagination. Pelican, Harmondsworth

Mocellin G 1995 Occupational therapy: a critical overview, part 1. British Journal of Occupational Therapy 58(12): 502–506

Mocellin G 1996 Occupational therapy: a critical overview, part 2. British Journal of Occupational Therapy 59(1): 11–16

Oakley A 1974 Housewife. Allen Lane, London

Open University D283 1975 A glossary of sociological concepts. Open University Press, Milton Keynes

Ortner S 1974 Is female to male as nature is to culture? In: Rosaldo M Z , Lamphere L (eds) Women, culture and society. Stanford University Press, Stanford, CA

Reilly M 1962 Occupational therapy can be one of the great ideas of 20th century medicine. American Journal of Occupational Therapy 16(1): 1–9

Vander Zanden J 1979 Sociology. John Wiley, New York

Webber G 1996 Occupational therapy: a postmodernist perspective. British Journal of Occupational Therapy 58(10): 439–440

Wilcock A A 1993 Editorial. Occupational Science: Australia 1(1) 1

Yerxa E J 1993 Occupational science: a new source of power for participants in occupational therapy. Occupational Science: Australia 1(1): 3–10

3

Social research methods

R. K. Jones   Margaret Nicol

WHAT IS RESEARCH?

There are many definitions of research, some narrow, others broad. Put simply, research is the systematic investigation of a problem, area or issue and is undertaken to increase knowledge (Bailey 1997). Research has always had an important place within medicine, but it is only more recently that professions such as occupational therapy have recognized the necessity of undertaking the 'systematic investigation' of their work. In addition, because of the biopsychosocial nature of occupational therapy, there has been a recognition that as the research methods of the biological sciences are important, so too are the methods of the social sciences.

Activity 3.1
Talk to therapists who qualified more than 15 years ago. Find out how prominent a place research held in the curriculum when they were at college.

This chapter will not tell you how to do research; for that information, you need to consult a research textbook. Instead, this chapter aims to outline the philosophy underpinning different approaches to research and how they influence the selection of research methods. We will describe the use of research within sociology, paying particular emphasis to qualitative research methods. Examples from occupational therapy research will also be used to illustrate the ways in which therapists have used various research techniques.

PHILOSOPHICAL UNDERPINNING OF RESEARCH METHODOLOGIES

All research methods are reflections of a philosophical or theoretical position, and, like Alice in Wonderland, we must begin at the beginning. The problem was concisely presented by Schultz nearly half a century ago when he stated that there were two major schools of thought when it comes to research methodologies (Box 3.1).

Box 3.1   Research methodologies

One [school of thought] holds that the methods of the natural sciences which have brought about such magnificent results are the only ones and that they alone, therefore, have to be applied in their entirety to the study of human affairs … The other school of thought feels that there is a basic difference in the structure of the social world and the world of nature. (Schultz 1976)

The problem that Schultz identified was basically that the methodology practised by the natural sciences was at variance with that of the social sciences because the subject matter itself was so totally different, the former being concerned with inanimate matter, the latter with conscious interactive behaviour. This difference has led to the categorization of research into two broad types:

1. positivist, also referred to as scientific or quantitative
2. qualitative, also referred to as interpretavist, and incorporating ethnography and phenomenology.

The particular approach adopted will influence how an investigation is undertaken, that is to say, the methodology and methods used. Jones (1993) provides a useful way of remembering the difference between methodology and methods. He describes methodology as being like the gardener's overall strategy for his or her garden (what to plant, what fertilizer to use, etc.). Methods, on the other hand, are like the particular tools the gardener uses (watering can, hoe and so on).

Before looking at qualitative research, we need

to understand what was for a long time the dominant research methodology – positivism.

POSITIVISM

The theoretical position known as positivism is thought to have originated with Auguste Comte (1798–1857), who viewed social life as being modelled on the physical world. Comte's belief that society was made up of laws similar to those of physical science was part of the process of reconstructionism that was gathering momentum at that time, i.e. the belief that society could be reconstructed according to scientific principles. Positivism is generally agreed as possessing the characteristics identified in Box 3.2.

Box 3.2   Characteristics of positivism

- Direct observation and definition of 'variables' results in the development of an 'hypothesis'
- This hypothesis can be tested by gathering measurable (quantitative) evidence
- Empirically valid statements are made, which can be tested against the quantitative data

---

Comte argued for the primacy of objective social structures. These 'social structures' are there when we are born, and we internalize them as part of the socialization process, learning them as cultural determinants of behaviour. Later, Emile Durkheim (1858–1917) held that the world was constituted of 'social facts' that are distinct from the concerns of biology and psychology. Early in the twentieth century, the logical positivists of the Vienna circle consolidated a 'hardline' positivism, which, through the 'verification principle', proposed that knowledge must, to be valid, be verifiable by sensory experience. Often this is via statistics and public records, for example counting the number of suicides and comparing the rates over time and with place. The consequence of this approach is that positivism espouses a quantitative methodology: objective facts must be measured objectively, as summarized in Box 3.2.

In summary, quantitative methodology implements the theoretical basis of positivism by claiming the following:

- There is a scientific basis to social behaviour.
- 'Measurement' forms the basis of ascertaining the nature of social order and human behaviour.
- If we can control the variables, we can gain an accurate 'picture' of the world.

There are different types of quantitative research methods, often categorized as follows:

- experimental designs
- quasi-experimental designs
- non-experimental designs.

For a fuller discussion of these methods, readers are referred to popular research texts such as Bailey (1997) or Depoy & Gitlin (1993), used by therapists.

Limitations of positivism

Positivism has been exposed to a number of criticisms, for example: Why is experience a sound basis for scientific knowledge?, why should science deal only with observable phenomena?, why should we distinguish between 'fact' and 'value'? (Blaikie 1993).

There are obvious problems with the positivist approach when trying to experiment in a scientific way with human beings:

- It is hardly ever feasible to conduct experiments on human beings, and when this is done, it is on a very small scale and extremely specific.
- It generally means removing the objects of study from their natural settings.
- By making human beings the object of study, we introduce the 'observer effect'; i.e. people, unlike rocks or rats, may change what they do because they know they are being observed in a test situation.

In terms of social science methodology, quantification is viewed as failing to grasp the essential nature of the social world by reducing it to a statistical simplicity. Complex social phenomena dealing with 'motive', 'meaning', etc. cannot be reduced to a single entity encapsulated in questionnaire analysis. The case of public records offers a good illustration. Government statistics and public records are generally regarded as sacrosanct, but on analysis, they are the result of human compilation and consequently open to error and misinterpretation.

As a result of these concerns and a belief that human beings are all unique and have differing experiences, another type of research method developed. This approach is antipositivist and sometimes known as qualitative, naturalistic or ethnographic research.

ANTIPOSITIVISM

Antipositivism originates from a different philosophical position from that of Comte. At the turn of the twentieth century, Max Weber (1864–1920) came to the conclusion that there were no 'social facts', while in America, W. I. Thomas (1863–1947) wrote about the 'definition of the situation' and argued that if people believe a situation to be real, this belief will shape their actions. Also within this tradition is G. H. Mead (1863–1931), who arrived at a philosophy of 'the self' emphasizing the way in which people reflect on how others see them and alter their behaviour accordingly.

There are some important differences between theorists in this tradition, but the main tenets of anti-positivism can be summarized as follows.

Human beings create material and non-material products, by which is meant everything around us that sociologists call culture, from a squash racquet (material product) to teenagers (non-material product). These cultural creations become part of what we term reality, even though they only exist because we have created them. Although we assimilate our culture through the process known as socialization, we are also able to change and develop that culture.

In antipositivism the individual is central. There is me, you, us and the words we share. There is also the vocabulary of non-verbal communication. That is to say, we 'understand' and communicate through non-verbal signals such as the way we dress and even the way we walk. Antipositivist methodologists believe that, as a result of what has been said above, research must be focused on the way in which the individual experiences the world. They subscribe to a 'dialectical developmentalism', which means that the very act of reflection is changing you, me and us.

Antipositivist, or qualitative, research is therefore concerned with what is termed an 'emic' perspective: understanding life from the participant's viewpoint within his or her natural environment. Polgar & Thomas (1995, p. 109) suggest that this type of research examines 'the personal meanings of individuals' experiences and actions in the context of their social environments'. There are a variety of qualitative research designs but, for the purposes of this text, only two major designs – ethnography and phenomenology – which have more direct relevance to occupational therapists, will be dealt with. For a more in-depth discussion of the full range of qualitative designs, readers are referred to Denzin & Lincoln (1994).

People who subscribe to this perspective share a common concern with investigating social behaviour where it naturally occurs, hence the term 'naturalistic' research. Another term that is often used to describe this fieldwork is ethnography.

Ethnography

Ethnography originated within anthropology and is broadly defined as the description of culture. It aims to understand a way of life from the participants' viewpoint and thus involves researchers becoming immersed in the object of their study, whether that is a hospital or a housing project. A range of data collection methods, including participant observation, interviewing and critically reviewing documents/records, are used to enable this to happen. It involves learning from people as well as learning about them.

Phenomenology

Phenomenology stems from the philosophy of Edmund Husserl (1859–1938) and starts with the idea that we can only know what we experience and that we understand the world on the basis of our experience. The adoption of this philosophy as a basis for investigating the social world underpins ethnomethodology and social constructionism.

Ethnomethodology

This particular approach is associated with the American sociologist Howard Garfinkel. Ethnomethodology is the translation of phenomenology into a research approach in the social sciences. The researcher is interested in the answer to the question 'What it is like to have certain experiences?' from the participants' perspective and to discover how they make sense of the world. This focus on how individuals understand the nature of the social action in which they are engaged leads to the in-depth exploration of small-scale interactions. This very often involves detailed analysis of videotapes or transcripts of conversations. For ethnomethodologists, one of the easiest ways of studying something is to look at what happens when situations break down. For example, it is only when we come across people with poor social skills that we become aware of the complex rules, such as those of turn-taking, governing our everyday conversations.

Activity 3.2

Tape-record and transcribe an informal 10-minute conversation between two or three of your friends.

You may notice, when you look at the results of the above activity, that what people actually say makes little grammatical sense: people finish each other's sentences, repeat what has been said and appear to 'get' what the person is saying before they have even finished. It looks chaotic, yet when you think back, it probably seemed very ordered and natural at the time. This illustrates the point made by ethnomethodologists that people actively work at making sense of and maintaining social interactions. They share a common understanding of the situation and act accordingly.

Some sociologists argue that we not only work at making sense of the world, but are also engaged in building it. This perspective is known as social constructionism.

Social constructionism

This approach stems from the work of Berger & Luckman (1967). Broadly speaking, social constructionism is the assumption not only that we live, for the most part, in 'different sub-universes of meaning', but that we also sustain these 'universes' with appropriate 'plausibility structures'. This seems very difficult to follow at first but becomes clearer when we look at the social construction of illness.

To say that illness is socially constructed means that it is given meaning both within cultures (different beliefs about what constitutes 'being ill' between varying social classes) and between cultures (the different health beliefs of a Xhosa tribesman and a Hollywood actor, for example) and over time (the way in which we think about what are now termed psychiatric conditions is different from the view of people in the sixteenth century). Illness does not exist *per se* but is the result of human social definitions.

Thus when researching issues concerning health and illness, Britten & Fisher (1993) stressed the importance of understanding the respondents' rather than the researchers' meanings, of concentrating on the individual rather than the population, and of trying to understand the way in which individuals construct their world, to minimize the researcher's intrusion and to attempt to understand the respondent's understanding of common terms. When we ask people whether they feel healthy at the moment, we first need to check what 'being healthy' means to them. Does it mean being at the peak of physical fitness or simply not being actively sick?

Antipositivist research

The main features of antipositivist research are summarized in Box 3.3.

A qualitative research strategy of the social

Box 3.3 Features of antipositivist research

- Social phenomena have to be understood through trying to establish people's perceptions and interpretations manifested through interactions. The process of talk (or language) is important here
- The nature of 'reality' is problematic, and what people really think about situations and events are not surface interpretations but a complexity of meanings and constructions
- People are not passive recipients of social forces but actively engage in the creation of the world around them

---

constructionist sort involves several common features:

1. The focus is on meanings and the attempt to understand the culture of those being studied, as far as possible in their natural settings. This suggests, for example, a preference for participant observation or observation rather than experiments under artificial conditions, and a preference for informal and less standardized interviews rather than more standardized formal ones.
2. Rather than testing preconceived hypotheses, such research aims to generate hypotheses and theories from the data that emerge, thus implying a greater degree of flexibility concerning research design and data collection and that the process of analysis occurs simultaneously with the process of data collection.
3. By focusing on social interaction, qualitative research involves the ongoing collection of data rather than sampling at discrete points (as with ticks on a questionnaire or interview schedule).
4. Qualitative research is holistic in the sense that it attempts to provide a contextual understanding of the complex interrelationships of causes and consequences that affect human behaviour and in so doing often incorporates a wide variety of specific research techniques, even within one research topic.

More phenomenologically orientated methodology is not without its critics or limitations. For example, such research is claimed to be too narrowly focused. A conversational analysis of the 'initial interview' situation between therapist and client seems to ignore the very real influence and constraints on people's lives of structural forces such as socioeconomic class and power. In addition, interpretavist researchers must subject their own claims to have discovered something to the same scepticism they apply to positivist claims to have established some fact. As a result of the perceived need to engage in research that is of immediate and practical value – particularly in the health- and social care field – a pragmatic approach has been developed.

RECENT DEVELOPMENTS IN THEORY AND PRACTICE

There have been a number of attempts to combine different methodologies and methods. Newby's *The deferential worker* (1977), for example, used census statistics, the survey and participant observation, while Barker's *Making of a Moonie: choice or brainwashing?* (1986) used the in-depth interview, participant observation and the questionnaire. This combination of methods and theories is called triangulation. If we look at an issue one way and then another, and if the results of both investigations are compatible, we can have a high degree of faith in our findings.

Contemporary research in the health- and social care field tends toward a combination of some of the features of interpretivism and positivism, and utilizes methods from both areas. There is an attempt to understand the 'external' mechanisms that shape social phenomena while at the same time being sympathetic to people's interpretation of the world. Social phenomena are perceived as being both produced and reproduced by members of society. This approach concentrates on wider forces in society and posits that phenomena can be explained by 'forces' other than those directly observable or thought to be involved. Thus the institutional elements in society actually combine and influence interactions, and social interactions can in turn in-

fluence the former (such as the political, religious and economic systems). There is an acceptance of the fact that various aspects of society may be such that we are unaware of them and they are in fact beyond our experience. The realist seeks the underlying causes of social phenomena, such as what the link between delinquency and family structure is, why a thing is as it is rather than another way, and how a belief is linked to a wider context. The realist tries, whenever possible, to use explanatory methods. Because realism assumes the independent existence of social reality, it also assumes that it can be observed and explained, consequently bridging the gap between micro and macro theory.

Mixing of approaches

Fetterman (1988) wrote:

One need only scratch the surface of the qualitative/quantitative debate to understand the terms 'quantitative' and 'qualitative' are in themselves misleading. They are commonly accepted handles for both the contrasting paradigms and the methods associated with them.

The mixing of approaches both increases our options and establishes that there are different interpretations of the same data.

It may be, as someone once said, only a matter of personal taste, but it is also closely linked with which particular paradigm we are intellectually committed to. The important consideration, even if it means employing a mix, is to arrive at an accurate description of the setting. The 'number-cruncher' approach rarely describes what goes on in the social setting of a school or of an occupational therapy department in a hospital, hence the gradual acceptance of qualitative research as an 'alternative' methodology. The blending of the two paradigms, however, rarely results in an equitable distribution of methodologies because of epistemological predispositions. However, the important message for all researchers is to select an appropriate method to fit the research question being asked and to consider both qualitative and quantitative methods as tools for the job. Morse & Field (1996, p. 3) endorse this view by stating, 'Smart researchers are adept at both qualitative and quantitative methods, and they use the appropriate method at the appropriate time, according to the type of research question, the goal of the research and other considerations.'

Research in the real world is also influenced by the fact that large-scale studies need funding. The people who fund the research may have a bias towards a certain type of methodology or to certain methods because of their relative cost. Thus questionnaires can be cheaper and quicker than participant observation carried out over a long period of time.

RESEARCH METHODS

There are several methods of data collection within qualitative research methods, the following being the main types.

Participant observation

This is one of the main ways in which sociologists gather primary data in qualitative methodology. It can be highly structured or diffuse, but above all it demands first-hand involvement in the social world. Its aim is to experience reality as the participants do by spending time in the setting, learning about daily life.

Morse & Field (1996), two nurses who write extensively about qualitative methods, have described four types of participant observation. Complete participation is where the researcher becomes a member of the culture being studied and conceals from the participants his or her identity as a researcher. With the participant-as-observer role, participants are aware of the role of the researcher, who spends time collecting data while carrying out a role within the group. The observer-as-participant role has as the researcher's main tasks interviewing and observing without having any function within the group. Finally, there is the observer role, in which the researcher is totally passive and has no interaction within the culture, perhaps viewing participants from behind a one-way mirror.

Thus the degree of participation is on a continuum, i.e. how far researchers involve themselves in the settings. So, also, is the degree of 'revealedness', i.e. how far the participants know that there is a study in progress. This raises problems of covert research, which has been criticized on the grounds of ethics. Two other problems are how intense the observation will be and how extensive. A final question concerns whether the focus of the study is specific or diffuse. Well-known examples of this method include Becker's (1963) *Boys in white* (a study of medical students) and Goffman's (1968) *Asylums* (a study of various institutions). The recording of observations and fieldnotes are essential in this type of research.

Interviews

Interviewing style varies within qualitative research. The unstructured interview is used when the researcher knows very little about the topic and is learning as the interview progresses. There are few specific questions, and the interviewee guides the interview, the main task of the interviewer being to listen. The semistructured interview is where the interviewer has an idea of the appropriate questions to ask but does not know the answers. The interviewer has a range of topics that he or she wishes to cover but does this in a flexible way, interviewees being encouraged to answer them in their own way. Morse & Field (1996) suggest that 'a successful qualitative interview is more like an intimate and personal sharing of a confidence with a trusted friend, and the information given must be treated likewise, with respect.'

In addition to the main methods of data collection outlined above, there are other methods that are being increasingly used in small-scale health research. Films, photographs and videotapes can often graphically capture the life of the group under study. Critical analysis of contemporary and historical records (newspapers, government documents, letters, or folklore) can also provide valuable data. Diaries can provide information on the day-to-day life of individuals and, although a relatively new technique within health research, can provide valuable insights.

VALIDITY AND ETHICS OF QUALITATIVE RESEARCH

Traditionally, antipositivist research, with its emphasis on interpretation, has been viewed by the medical establishment as suspect in terms of its validity. Such research is not amenable to the use of control groups, statistical analysis and statements of probability, which have been considered the norm. However, taken-for-granted 'hard' data such as birthweight (Oakley 1991) and suicide rates have also recently been viewed as 'subjective', i.e. as part of a social process that allows human error and subjectivism to enter the area.

The debate about the validity of results is now less of an issue, qualitative research being more broadly accepted. The area currently considered to be most problematic is that of ethics. A collection of ethically 'tricky' research programmes, most of which come under the label of 'qualitative' methodologies, are discussed by Bulmer (1982). How are we to view the eight sane people who gained admission to 12 different hospitals in order to study the psychiatrically ill (Rosenhan 1973)? Or the social scientist who observed hundreds of homosexual acts in public lavatories in America (Humphreys 1970)? The main arguments used against covert or hidden research include that such research violates the principle of informed consent, that it is an invasion of personal privacy and that deception is invariably involved. Nevertheless, well-known social scientists, such as Festinger, Garfinkel, Goffman and, Bulmer, have utilized it, and we have been able to gain access to such areas as criminal abortion, the social life of a school and 'deviant' sexuality.

Activity 3.3

How would you feel if you found out that a member of your group was not really a student but a researcher looking at how to become an occupational therapist?

Of course, research in the medical field has always been subject to more (although not always much more) scrutiny than has that carried out by sociologists. Nevertheless, there are still important questions to be considered. A particular issue being raised by disabled people is the question of who decides which questions are to be researched, what the role of those being researched is and who gets to find out about the results of the research (French & Swain 1997). Disabled people have called for the development of participatory research (i.e. that which directly involves people in the research process) and emancipatory research (i.e. that which leads to the removal of barriers that disabled people face). This is an important question for occupational therapists and will be returned to later.

RESEARCH AND THE OCCUPATIONAL THERAPIST

Some of the research in which occupational therapists are engaged requires a clearly scientific or positivist approach, for example if one is carrying out an evaluation of a new type of pressure-relief cushion or wants to know whether a resting splint prevents joint deformity. In these cases, some form of experimental design would be highly appropriate. On the other hand, research aiming to find out why people do not use recommended equipment could use a questionnaire, although much richer data are likely to be gained using interviews.

Positivist research does have its uses for occupational therapists, not least because the people who purchase occupational therapy (government agencies, insurance companies, etc.) tend to prefer 'hard' quantitative data. However, therapists have also developed an interest in more antipositivist approaches, particularly when investigating predominantly sociological questions such as what is the nature of occupation and how do organizations influence the way in which we practise?

Activity 3.4

Compare and contrast the methodologies and methods used in research articles found in your own professional journal with those of other professions such as social work or physiotherapy.

ETHNOGRAPHIC APPROACHES WITHIN OCCUPATIONAL THERAPY

Krefting (1989), an occupational therapist, makes a very good case for why occupational therapists should use ethnography, coining the phrase 'disability ethnography'. Townsend, in a more recent study (1996), used institutional ethnography to illustrate occupational therapy's mental health practice. This study utilized observation, interviews and document reviews as the primary data collection methods. Townsend collected data in seven adult mental health day settings in different parts of Canada over a 6-month period. She found that occupational therapists work on empowering individuals through the use of occupations. However, when these occupations are viewed within the overall context of case management, they tend to be negated and 'made to fit prevailing medical and psychological ideas about health'. The investigation uncovered the way in which the 'culture' of the organization gets in the way of therapists practising in the way they would like. This study is a good example of a therapist explicitly using a sociological approach to examine practice.

PHENOMENOLOGICAL APPROACHES WITHIN OCCUPATIONAL THERAPY

Hasselkus & Dickie (1994) used phenomenology to understand the nature of the experience of 'doing' occupational therapy. In their study, they were interested in gaining an understanding of satisfying and dissatisfying occupational therapy. In order to do this, they sampled 200 occupational therapists and obtained data from 148 respondents. The data were initially collected by a written questionnaire. The main phenomenological questions were posed as follows:

think back over your practice as an occupational therapist and identify one incident or case when you felt especially satisfied (dissatisfied) with the occupational therapy that you provided. Describe that case, including what you did, why you did it, what the outcome was, what was most satisfying (dissatisfying) to you.

The questionnaire is not a research tool well

suited to a phenomenological approach and, perhaps unsurprisingly, produced only 24 completed responses. This required the researchers to reconsider their data collection method; they then conducted telephone interviews with the 123 other respondents. In analysing the data, Hasselkus & Dickie, in their detailed discussion concluded that there were three overarching dimensions of practice, which they labelled change, community and craft. 'Change' related to the outcome of the case, the inability to make any difference being overall the most telling theme of dissatisfaction. 'Community' was described as the interpersonal or relationship aspects. The craft dimension focused on what the therapist did and in many cases identified the complex strands the occupational therapists had to manage, reaffirming the holistic nature of the intervention.

Activity 3.5

Do you see any weaknesses in using the telephone to collect data about the way in which people experience their world?

Although one may wish to question whether telephone, as opposed to person-to-person, interviews are the best strategy for collecting rich data, this was still a useful study. In this instance, the phenomenological approach enabled the researchers to abstract from individual therapists' experiences three generalizable constructs or categories of experience. These constructs could be used as a basis for further investigation and employed in the analyses of other examples of therapists engaged in or talking about their practice. A similar, more classical phenomenological approach has been used by McLaughlin Gray (1997) to examine the concept of occupation.

PARTICIPATORY AND EMANCIPATORY RESEARCH

Occupational therapists are no exception to the rule that health professionals tend to do research 'on' people in attempt to answer questions that professionals themselves think are important. This is not to say that research of value to disabled people has not been carried out. However, it is important that we respond to the demands articulated by French & Swain (1997), as outlined above.

In Canada, Townsend (1997) describes how, through her work with users of mental health services, some of these issues are beginning to be addressed. She and other professionals have been involved in giving service users research skills that they can then apply to questions of personal importance. However, Townsend also highlights some of the structural barriers to the development of projects such as this, for example limited access to funding and the lack of accepted research qualifications that research funding agencies or conference paper reviewers may expect. People who hold the title 'researcher' have status and power; service users do not.

CONCLUSION

Sociologists have used a variety of research methodologies and methods. We have seen how the early positivist approach gave way, under the strain of great criticism, to more ethnographic and phenomenological approaches. More recently, there has been a recognition of the value of taking a mixed approach, particularly in relation to research in health and social care. Quantitative research can, for example, highlight that people from lower socioeconomic classes suffer more ill-health; qualitative approaches can help us look at people's experience of this.

Occupational therapists are also becoming aware of the value of antipositivist research approaches. In particular, ethnographic and phenomenological methodologies are helpful when exploring the nature of occupation and issues such as client-centred practice. Finally, research by therapists has always been subject to ethical review procedures. These procedures have, however, not necessarily considered the issue of the participation or emancipation of disabled people.

REFERENCES

Bailey D 1997 Research for the health professional, 2nd edn. F A Davies, Philadelphia

Barker E 1986 Making of a Moonie: choice or brainwashing? Blackwell, Oxford

Becker H 1963 Boys in white. Chicago University Press, Chicago

Berger P, Luckman T 1967 The social construction of reality. Allen Lane The Penguin Press, London

Blaikie N 1993 Approaches to social enquiry. Polity Press, Cambridge

Britten N, Fisher B 1993 Qualitative research and general practice. British Journal of General Practice 43(372): 270–271

Bulmer M 1982 Social research ethics. Macmillan, London

Denzin N K, Lincoln Y S 1994 Handbook of qualitative research. Sage, Thousand Oaks, CA

Depoy E, Gitlin L N 1993 Introduction to research. C V Mosby, St Louis

Fetterman D M 1988 A qualitative shift in allegiance. In: Fetterman D M (ed.). Qualitative approaches to evaluation in education: the silent scientific revolution. Praeger, New York

French S, Swain J 1997 Changing disability research: participating and emancipatory research with disabled people. Physiotherapy 83(1): 26–32

Goffman E 1968 Asylums. Penguin, Harmondsworth

G J McLaughlin Gray 1997 Application of the phenomenological method to the concept of occupation. Journal of Occupational Science (Australia) 4(1): 5–17

Hasselkus B R, Dickie V A 1994 Doing occupational therapy: dimensions of satisfaction and dissatisfaction. American Journal of Occupational Therapy 48(2): 145–154

Humphreys L 1970 Tearoom trade: impersonal sex in public places. Aldine, Chicago

Jones P 1993 Studying society: sociological theories and research practices. Collins Educational, London

Krefting L 1989 Disability ethnography: a methodological approach for occupational therapy research. Canadian Journal of Occupational Therapy 56(2): 61–66

Morse J M, Field P A 1996 Nursing research, 2nd edn. Chapman & Hall, London

Newby H 1977 The deferential worker. Allen Lane, London

Oakley A 1991 Times Higher Educational Supplement 28 October: 2

Polgar S, Thomas S A 1995 Introduction to research in the health sciences, 3rd edn. Churchill Livingstone, Edinburgh

Rosenhan D L 1973 On being sane in insane places. Science 179: 250–259

Schultz A 1976 The phenomenology of the social world. Heinemann, London

Townsend E 1996 Enabling empowerment: using simulations versus real occupations. Canadian Journal of Occupational Therapy 63(2): 114–128

Townsend E 1997 Occupation: potential for personal and social transformation. Journal of Occupational Science (Australia) 4(1): 18–26

CHAPTER CONTENTS

4

Social stratification and social class

T. Hartery   T. Gahagan

WHY STUDY SOCIAL STRATIFICATION?

Social stratification is important for a number of reasons. To begin with, every aspect of a person's life, whether or not they realize it, is affected by stratification. What kind of education they receive, whom they marry, their health status, how long they live and even their likelihood of going to prison are dependent on their position in the stratification system. Social stratification also presents groups with different experiences and problems that can lead them to develop their own subcultures, as well as some awareness of common interests and a common identity. This awareness of common interests and identity, together with tensions between groups over inequalities, can lead to conflict and change in a society.

The existence of these differences between people has particular implications for occupational therapists. In the latter part of this chapter, we will look at the position of therapists in the social stratification system and pay particular attention to the issue of inequalities in health between different groups.

SOCIAL STRATIFICATION

Sociologists use the term 'social stratification' to describe the division of society into unequal groups, although such inequality is more complex than being simply differences in the amount of money that people have. Social stratification usually has three different components (Bilton et al 1987):

1. inequalities in life chances: some groups have higher levels of material advantages than others, for example greater wealth and income, better health and education or greater job security
2. inequalities in status: certain groups in society claim and receive higher levels of status, prestige or social honour than other groups; status differences may rest on such things as level of income, occupation and skin colour
3. inequalities in power: some groups are in a better position to control or influence other groups.

These three dimensions of stratification usually go together, so that certain groups are persistently advantaged in terms of life chances, status and power while other groups are persistently disadvantaged. In industrial societies, for example, the heads of leading companies are likely to earn a high income, be respected by the community and have power over many people and concerns. By way of contrast, the unemployed are poor, of low status and lacking in power.

Stratification as structured inequality

The fact that inequalities are distributed in this manner leads on to the idea of stratification as structured inequality. This means that inequalities are not regarded by sociologists as random or haphazard occurrences. Rather, they arise out of the relationship between social groups, are distributed in the ways described above and tend to persist over generations. In relation to this last point, for example, Westergaard & Resler (1976) state that, as far as Britain is concerned, 'despite progressive changes to the tax system, the retention of a massive share of all wealth by the top 5 or 10% of the population is very striking.'

If stratification is structured inequality, the question arises of why stratification exists in the first place. While more detailed explanations for this must wait until later in the chapter, the basic answer is that stratification arises as a means of regulating access to scarce resources

in a society (Worsley 1977). It emerges because one group has a monopoly of some resource that allows them to control the distribution of rewards and to claim the larger share for themselves. What that 'something' is has varied historically. In preindustrial societies, it has included physical force and claims by priests to exclusive contact with supernatural forces (Hurd et al 1973). In modern industrial societies, the monopoly ownership of the means of production has been cited by several sociologists as being the major cause of stratification.

Once established, stratification systems tend to persist because privileged groups take steps to maintain their privileges. They may, for example, gain political power and pass laws backed up by the threat or use of force to protect their privilege. The Apartheid regime in South Africa was a clear example of this, as whites sought to maintain their position relative to blacks. Another mechanism is the ability of privileged groups to buy the best education for their children, thus helping to ensure that they are able to maintain their parents' position.

Activity 4.1

Do you think that the division of society into those who have and those who have not is inevitable or a good thing?

Class stratification

Historically, there have been several different types of stratification system, for example caste and age-set stratification and feudalism (Box 4.1). Western industrial societies, however, are stratified by social class. Giddens (1992) defines a class as a 'a large-scale grouping of people who share common economic resources which strongly influence the type of lifestyle they are able to lead' and argues that Western societies are divided into three social classes: an upper class of wealth-holders, a middle class of professionals and white collar workers, and a working class of manual workers. While the implication of this is that such societies are highly unequal, one problem is that sociologists do not agree on a definition of

---

Box 4.1 Different types of stratification system

- *Caste*: closed status groups in which an individual's position in the status hierarchy is fixed by birth. Members of the highest castes have greater wealth and power than those in lower castes
- *Age-set*: status groups the membership of which is determined by age. In age-set societies, the elderly form the age-set with the highest status and the young that with the lowest. However, status is not fixed, as in a caste system, but increases as the people in a particular age-set grow older
- *Feudalism*: a system that existed in medieval Europe and consisted of four strata: the nobility, who, through their military power, were able to gain control over much of the land; the clergy, who also had access to land; the burgesses, who acquired wealth through trade; and the serfs, who cultivated the land for the nobility and clergy

---

social class, how many classes there are or even why class exists. In order to clarify this situation, it is necessary to look at a number of theories and models.

Marx on social class

Karl Marx (1818–83) argued that classes were groups who shared the same relationship to the forces of production. On this basis, he saw capitalist society as being divided into two main social classes: the bourgeoisie, or owners of the forces of production (factories, machines and raw materials), and the proletariat, or workers, who have to sell their labour to the bourgeoisie in order to live. The relationship between the classes was one of antagonism and conflict since the bourgeoisie used their ownership to exploit the workers, leading to poverty and oppression on the part of the workers. For Marx, therefore, it is the fact that the forces of production are owned by one class that is the crucial point in understanding class stratification.

The ownership of the forces of production gave the bourgeoisie political as well as economic power. This followed because the bourgeoisie were able to get members of their own class into top positions in the state. Thus, according to Marx, not only the government, but also the judiciary, army and police were headed by members of

that class. This meant that these state institutions worked in the interests of the bourgeoisie. From Marx's perspective, then, the owning class was also the ruling class.

Marx went on to argue that certain features in the development of capitalism (for example the crisis of overproduction, the pauperization of the working class and a growing polarization between classes) would inevitably lead to the overthrow of capitalism and the establishment of a Communist society in which private property would disappear. In such a society, the principle of production and distribution would be 'from each according to his ability, to each according to his need'. Before this can happen, however, the proletariat needs to change from a class 'in itself' to a class 'for itself'.

Marx thus uses the term 'class' in two ways. In the early stages of capitalism, he recognizes that, while the proletariat occupy a common economic position (as non-owners of the forces of production), they may have little awareness of themselves as a class with a common identity and similar problems. However, as capitalism develops and capitalist exploitation increases, the proletariat will develop a revolutionary class consciousness that will lead them to view themselves as a group with a common identity, common problems and common goals. When this class consciousness is established, the proletariat will change from a class in itself to a class for itself, in Marx's terms a class proper.

To be a class proper, an economic group must have some degree of class consciousness, some notion of its identity compared with that of other groups, together with elements of a common culture and a desire and willingness to pursue class interests against the interests of other classes. In a true class system, therefore, people will describe and think about themselves and others in class terms and act on that basis, for example joining political parties that express their class interests, following leisure activities

---

Activity 4.2

Do laws tend to favour employers or employees?

that are class based and living their lives on the basis of specific class norms and values (the idea of classes as subcultures will be developed later in the chapter).

Weber and class

Max Weber (1864–1920) agreed with Marx that capitalist society was dominated by an owning class but argued that Marx's two-class model was unrealistic when industrialization had given rise to so many new occupations. Instead, he saw four social classes and defined a class as a group who share a similar level of life chances because of a common market situation. The notion of market situation reflects the fact that only a small proportion of people own the forces of production while the majority are non-owners who have to sell their labour to employers in order to live. Some occupational groups in this position have more favourable market situations than others, meaning that their skills are more in demand by employers or that they are in short supply. As a result, they receive a higher level of life chances (more money, greater job security and perks such as company cars) and thus belong to a higher class. Occupational groups with less favourable market situations (who are less in demand by employers or exist in larger numbers) receive fewer benefits from the labour market so belong to a lower class. For Weber, then, market position equalled class position.

On the basis of market situation, Weber saw four classes in modern society, class 1 having the highest level of life chances and class 4 the lowest (Box 4.2).

Status stratification

According to Weber, class was only one basis for stratification. In addition, he saw stratification by

---

Box 4.2   Weber's social classes

1. A dominant ownership and commercial class
2. White collar workers and the intelligentsia
3. The petty bourgeoisie, i.e. small shop owners
4. The manual working class

Activity 4.3

Which of the following have the most and least favourable market situations?

Typist	Lawyer
Nurse	Road sweeper
Business executive	Occupational therapist
Labourer	Teacher

---

status. Status stratification refers to the division of society into a status hierarchy, each status group viewing members of its own group as equals and those of other groups as inferiors or superiors. In this hierarchy, status is determined by such things as occupation, education, income, accent and, crucially, style of life (how people live, especially what consumer goods they have). Those at the top of the status system have status attributes, including a lifestyle, that other groups regard as superior to their own. As a result, they demand and receive the deference and respect of other groups, who in turn often seek to copy the lifestyle and manners of this top-status group. In a status system, then, emulation and competition for status are the dominant social processes, compared with conflict in a class system.

Activity 4.4

What are the attributes of a high- and a low-status position in your country?

In reality, class and status usually go together, since high income is usually necessary for a high-status lifestyle. That means that people in a high class position are often the ones with the highest status as well. It also means that, in everyday usage, the terms 'class' and 'status' are used interchangeably. However, Weber argued that status was not reducible to class (thus differing from Marx, who saw status as an automatic accompaniment of high social class) and that, in certain situations, a person's class and status positions may be different. An example of this would be an aristocrat found guilty of a criminal offence or a dustman who is also a local councillor.

The status system can affect the class system

in a number of ways, especially in relation to class formation and class action. While class action requires a sense of class identity before it can occur, status divisions within a class can prevent its members feeling the sense of solidarity necessary for such action. An example here might be if white manual workers felt superior to black workers and discriminated against them on that basis. In addition, the fact that the highest classes usually have the highest status may serve to justify class inequalities and thus reduce the likelihood of class conflict.

Bringing together Marx and Weber

Bilton et al (1987) argue that elements of Marx and Weber can be combined to produce a three-class model of Western industrial societies. At the top of the class structure is a small but wealthy upper class, similar to Marx's bourgeoisie, who own the forces of production, while differences in market capacity (or market situation) give rise to a middle class of non-manual workers and a working class of manual workers. Beneath the working class are 'the poor' – the disabled, lone-parent families, the long-term unemployed, etc. – who have the lowest level of life chances because of their marginal or non-existent market situation.

Registrar-General's classification of social classes

So far, the idea of class has been dealt with theoretically in order to give some understanding of the nature of a class society. What these theories and models do not do, except in very general terms, is give some idea of who is in each class. For this purpose in Britain, the Registrar-General's classification of social classes is often used. Using occupation as an indicator of class, the Registrar-General views classes as groupings of people with broadly similar levels of occupational skill and status who also share similar living standards and ways of life. The notion of social classes sharing similar living standards and ways of life follows from the fact that occupation correlates fairly well with other compo-

nents of social position such as education and income. On the basis of occupation, the Registrar-General sees British society as being divided into five social classes (Box 4.3).

Box 4.3 The Registrar-General's classification

1   Professional, e.g. lawyer, doctor, top civil servant
2   Intermediate, e.g. teacher, nurse, manager
3N Skilled non-manual, e.g. typist, clerk, policeman
3M Skilled manual, e.g. miner, electrician, plumber
4   Semiskilled manual, e.g. bus conductor, farm-worker
5   Unskilled manual, e.g. labourer, cleaner

In this scheme, classes 1, 2 and 3N are broadly conceived of as the middle class, classes 3M, 4 and 5 being regarded as the working class

---

SOCIAL CLASSES AS SUBCULTURES

Many sociologists regard social classes as subcultures, with upper and middle-class groups to some extent having different norms and values from the working class. Lockwood (1966), for example, described the subculture of one working-class group, the proletarian traditionalists. While this study cannot be applied to the working class as a whole, it does provide some evidence for the idea of classes as subcultures.

According to Lockwood, proletarian traditionalists are workers who work in long-established industries such as coal mining and who live in close-knit, working-class communities. Living and working together produces strong bonds between workers and leads to the development of particular subcultural norms and values. According to Lockwood, the proletarian traditionalist subculture tends to be fatalistic and present-time orientated. Fatalism means that individuals feel that there is little they can do to alter their situation and that what happens to them depends on luck or fate. Such an attitude discourages long-term planning and encourages a present orientation, meaning that such people tend to live for the present, do not plan for the future and seek immediate gratification rather than being willing to put off pleasure now in return for greater rewards in the future.

By way of contrast, middle-class subculture is characterized by a sense of control over one's destiny and the idea that individuals can influence what happens to them through their own efforts. This attitude is linked to a future-time orientation that involves an ability to plan for the future and the ability to defer gratification, to put off having pleasure now in order to gain greater rewards in the future (Haralambos & Holborn 1995).

CLASS INEQUALITIES IN BRITAIN

Britain is often held up to be the epitome of a class-dominated society. The idea that Britain has a class system is borne out by evidence on inequalities in wealth, income and health.

Inequalities in wealth

Wealth refers to marketable assets, i.e. things that can be sold for income, for example consumer goods such as cars or houses, land and stocks and shares. Wealth therefore seems to mean the same as property. A crucial distinction here is the difference between wealth in the form of productive property and wealth as consumption property (Bilton et al 1987). Productive property refers to assets such as land and shares, which yield massive unearned income to their owners in the form of rents and dividends from company profits. Consumption property, on the other hand, refers to houses, cars, videos and so on. While these can be sold for income, they do not earn unearned income for their possessor.

In Britain, privately owned wealth is very unequally divided. In 1991 the richest 1% of adults owned 18% of the wealth, with the richest 10% owning 50% (Inland Revenue figures). A similar situation obtains in America, where the richest 1% own about 20% of the nation's wealth (US Department of Commerce 1993). The more wealth owned, the higher the proportion held as productive property, all of which provides unearned income. The top 1% in Britain, for example, own about 75% of privately owned shares, with the top 5% owning over 90% of the total (HMSO figures 1992). Smaller wealth-holders tend to hold more of their wealth in consumption property, which does not provide such income.

The British upper class

The inequality in the ownership of wealth points to the existence of a small but immensely wealthy upper or capitalist class in Britain. This group, amounting to between 0.1 and 10% of the adult population, owns substantial amounts of productive wealth in the form of shares, land or both, from which they derive a massive unearned income. This group includes the major owners of the forces of production, the directors of many of the largest companies and those who live on inherited wealth. This group, numbering around 43 500 people, between them owned about 7% of the nation's wealth in 1986, each individual being worth a minimum of £740 000 (Scott 1991).

Inequalities in life chances between middle and working classes

The majority of people in Britain do not own large amounts of productive wealth and have to rely on their occupation as their main source of income. For these, following Weber, it is differences in market situation that determine their class position and level of life chances. On the basis of market situation, most sociologists still distinguish between a middle class of non-manual workers and a working class of manual workers, non-manual workers experiencing a higher level of life chances than manual workers.

Differences in life chances between these two groups can be seen in the area of income and employment. Manual workers not only receive on average considerably less than non-manual workers, but also have to work more hours per week to achieve a gross average weekly wage that is about 25% less than that of non-manual workers (Bilton et al 1987). In addition, it is suggested that non-manual workers have more job security, longer holidays, more fringe benefits and greater promotion prospects than manual workers. They also have better health and live longer, are more likely to own their own home and a range of consumer goods, and are less likely to be convicted of a criminal offence (Haralambos & Holborn 1995).

Social class and health

Another significant difference in life chances between the classes relates to their differing likelihood of being in good health. The Black Report (1982) (quoted in Townsend & Davidson 1988) presented clear evidence that health status was dependent on social class, classes 4 and 5 having worse health at each stage of life compared with the higher social classes.

Social class differences in mortality

Black's figures showed that, at birth and during the first month of life, the risk of death for the children of unskilled workers was double that found in professional families. For the next 11 months, the risk increased, three male children of unskilled parents dying for every one male child of professional parents. In the age range 1–13 years, similar statistics applied: for boys in class 5, the risk of death was twice that for boys in class 1. For adults (men aged 20–64, women aged 20–59), a similar picture emerged, those in class 5 being twice as likely to die before retirement than those in class 1.

Black's figures were updated by Whitehead (1988), the same relationship between class and health being clearly visible. Again, babies whose fathers were in social class 5 ran twice the risk of stillbirth and death under 1 year of age compared with babies whose fathers were in social class 1. Similarly, adults in social class 5 run twice the risk of death as those in class 1. In terms of cause of death, with a few exceptions, the lower social classes experience the full range of killer diseases to a greater extent than do higher classes.

Social class differences in morbidity

In addition to higher death rates, the lower social classes also experience more illness of a non-life-threatening kind compared with the higher social classes. In terms of limiting longstanding illness, for example, the rate for men and women in social class 5 is twice that of social class 1. When considering types of illness, the lower social classes have higher rates of many common diseases, such as bronchitis, arthritis/rheumatism and varicose veins. Their psychological health is also worse, as are their general fitness levels. It is in middle age that the differences between the classes is greatest. Thus there is little difference in illness rates up to the age of 45, but a steep gradient emerges for those aged 45–65 (Whitehead 1988).

A growing health divide

It is not just that inequalities in health exist between the social classes but that the gap has actually widened in the past few decades, especially for adults. Comparing death rates in men between 1949 and 1983, for example, shows that they have declined more rapidly in the higher social classes than in the lower, causing the health gap to increase. The one exception to this worsening trend is in relation to deaths in babies under 1 year of age, where great improvements have occurred, thus reducing the health gap in this age range (Whitehead 1988).

Explanations for class inequalities in health

In seeking to explain these statistics, Black examined four possible explanations for the relationship between class and health:

- artefact

- natural or social selection
- cultural/behavioural
- materialist/structuralist.

Artefact explanation

This argues that the relationship between class and health is artificial in that it is a product of the measuring process itself. Thus, where occupation is used as an indicator of class, this disguises the extent to which health inequalities are really the result of changes in the occupational structure rather than some aspect of social class (wealth, income, culture, etc.).

These occupational changes have caused classes 4 and 5 to contract and other classes to expand, the result being that older, less healthy men tend to remain in semi and unskilled jobs. The worse health record of classes 4 and 5 may therefore be the result of the greater age of these groups. This implies that the real relationship is between age and health, or occupation and health, rather than class and health. One argument against this view is that measurements of health that take account of the age differences between classes (standardized mortality rates) still show evidence of class differences in health.

Natural or social selection

This explanation accepts that a relationship exists between class and health but reverses the argument, stating that health determines class. Thus healthy higher-class people can maintain their class position, while healthy members of the lower class can rise up the class system. Similarly ill-health may cause higher-class people to drift down the class structure, while unhealthy lower class people will fail to reach their potential. Black argues that whereas there is some evidence to show that such selection does occur, it is on too small a scale adequately to explain the health inequalities that exist.

Cultural/behavioural explanation

This argues that individuals damage their own health through engaging in health-damaging behaviours such as smoking, unhealthy diet and a lack of exercise. In particular, this explanation is used to explain the poor health record of classes 4 and 5 since evidence shows that such behaviours are concentrated in these groups.

Social classes 4 and 5 are held to adopt these behaviours either because they are less educated or more feckless than other classes or because they live in communities where the norms encourage people to act in these ways. In either case, the cultural/behavioural explanation regards individuals as being responsible for their own ill-health, so is sometimes referred to as 'victim-blaming'.

Materialist/structuralist explanation

This argument contains a number of strands. One is that poverty or economic deprivation arising from the workings of the capitalist system is the main cause of the poor health of classes 4 and 5. Here, Black thought that low income, poor housing, poor diet and unemployment were all factors that might be linked, individually or in combination, with ill-health in classes 4 and 5. However, another part of the materialist argument is that classes 4 and 5 do work that is more dangerous or less fulfilling, or productive of more physical or mental strain, than that of those in classes 1 and 2.

The materialist explanation and health inequalities throughout the life cycle

Overall, Black felt that the materialist explanation provided the best general explanation for class differences in health, although he recognized that other explanations could to a limited extent be involved. The following examples show how the materialist explanation can be applied to health at different stages of life.

Deaths during infancy. The fact that social class 5 babies are twice as likely to die in the first year of life results, in particular, from the greater incidence of accidents and respiratory disease in this group. Black argues that it might be that low income prevents class 5 parents providing safe, warm, hygienic homes and interferes with their ability to provide continuous, loving care.

1–14 Years. Almost all the difference in mortality between class 1 and 5 is due to a higher incidence of accidents, respiratory disease and, to a lesser extent, congenital abnormalities in class 5 children.

Although cultural factors may be involved, the main reason is material. With accidents, for example, class 5 parents lack the income to buy property that provides a safe place for children to play, or their houses may be less safe through their inability to pay for repairs or maintain equipment. Also, it could be that the lack of resources and the higher level of stressful life events associated with this again affects parents, so that they are less able to provide continuous and vigilant care.

15–64 Year-olds (adults). The materialist explanation is held to apply to this age group for two main reasons. In terms of working conditions, we have already seen how Black argues that the nature of manual work means that classes 4 and 5 are more likely to die from accidents or long-term exposure to dust, dirt or poisonous substances. Although important, this explanation alone is not sufficient to explain the extent of health inequalities: the role of material deprivation also has to be considered. Here, Black is less certain on how poverty affects adult health but highlights the prevalence of smoking among manual groups as an important cause of ill-health. This may in turn reflect social and economic factors connected with a low class position. Later research has supported this conclusion, arguing that health-damaging behaviours such as smoking and poor diet need to be understood as a reaction to adverse material circumstances, for example a lack of resources, poor housing and unemployment (Graham 1987, Whitehead 1988). However, as we shall see later in this chapter, it is not just material disadvantage that is important, but also differences in power and control.

SOCIAL CLASS AND OCCUPATIONAL THERAPY

Social stratification and social class are not key words commonly encountered in any search of the occupational therapy literature. Despite this apparent gap, Kelly (1996) for one has hinted that social class has been an influence on the profession from the start. He reminds us that many of its founders were women from middle-class backgrounds. Despite this historical, and perhaps continuing, middle-class dominance of the profession, the relevance of social class has gone largely unexplored. The remainder of this chapter looks at the social class position of occupational therapists and tackles the issue of inequalities in health in relation to implications for practice.

Activity 4.7

Do you think that the profession is dominated by people from higher socioeconomic backgrounds?

CLASS POSITION OF OCCUPATIONAL THERAPISTS

Using approaches to stratification, such as that of the Registrar-General outlined above, occupational therapists are clearly identified as belonging to the middle classes. Not only is occupational therapy a middle class-profession, but, if we look at the background of people entering higher education, there is evidence, in England at least, that they are mostly from middle-class backgrounds. The Higher Education Funding Council for England reported that half of the young people living in the wealthiest neighbourhoods were likely to go to university, compared with one in 10 from the poorest areas (Times Higher Educational Supplement, 1997). This, of course, begs the question of whether this really matters; after all, occupational therapy claims to be a client-centred profession that considers the needs of the individual. To answer this question, it is helpful to review some of the material on class subcultures.

CLASS SUBCULTURES

We saw earlier in this chapter how studies such as those by Lockwood identified the existence of different class cultures. In the same vein,

Mosey (1986), an influential American therapist, notes that social class binds people together and produces an element of 'cultural understanding'. Some therapists have taken this notion on board and discussed the influence of social class in terms of its effect on behaviour.

Krefting & Krefting (1991) subscribe to the view that social class is relevant in determining how much individuals' behaviour is influenced by their class subculture. They state that people who are from a working-class background will be more influenced by their class position than those from the middle classes. Yelton & Neilson (1991) undertook case studies of two working-class people from the Southern Appalachian region in the USA and identified different cultural values at odds with the rest of white, middle-class America. They used these studies to highlight the importance for therapists of understanding these values rather than viewing behaviour in terms of their own values. Similarly, Robinson (1987) highlights the possibility of therapists viewing client behaviour through the 'cultural filter' of a white, middle-class background with all the values and expectations that go along with it. Chapparo & Ranka (1995) have questioned the extent to which therapists are able to uncouple their own values and perspectives to reach a full understanding of the client's situation.

This notion of people with similar class backgrounds sharing some kind of understanding needs to be treated with caution. Although two people might share a common class background, there may be other more important cultural differences, such as those of region, ethnic group or gender. For example, one might consider how much 'cultural understanding' there would be between a working-class woman from rural Northwest Scotland and a working-class Asian man from Glasgow. Thus there are many interconnected and interdependent influences acting on people.

Activity 4.8

What differences would you identify between people from different social classes in your area?

It follows from what has been said that when therapist and client share the same class background, they are likely to come to a better understanding more easily. Thus it is possible that social class is a factor in determining how well therapist and client understand each other and therefore work effectively together.

Activity 4.9

What is the social class mix of your year group and how does it compare with the majority of clients you come across on fieldwork placements?

INEQUALITIES IN HEALTH AND OCCUPATIONAL THERAPY

Occupational therapists are concerned with working with people to develop their occupational performance to a satisfactory level, as determined by the client. In order to do this, therapists need to inform themselves of the factors influencing the person's particular condition and his or her ability to achieve desired goals. It is at this level that the Black Report introduced earlier in this chapter has particular relevance to occupational therapists.

You will recall that the Black Report concluded that there is a strong relationship between poor health and social class. That is to say, people in lower socioeconomic groups have poorer living conditions (income, housing, etc.), which leads to an increase in illness and disability. The other main contending explanation for inequalities in health was the cultural/behavioural explanation, i.e. people engage in behaviours that are damaging to their health because they choose to or because of social factors. Acceptance of either of these explanations could have an impact on the way in which therapists practise.

Occupational therapy and the materialist/structuralist explanation

The Black Report highlighted that there is much evidence to suggest that poverty – a feature of life in the lower socioeconomic classes – is a major cause of ill-health. If this is the case, one may be led to conclude that therapists can have little impact, in the long term, on a person's well-being. What is the point, it could be argued, in rehabilitation if the person is discharged to living conditions that contributed to the problem in the first place. Paying for more therapists to work in a stroke unit, and thereby providing more rehabilitation, is of limited use if people are going back to social conditions, for example cold, damp housing, that may precipitate another stroke. For governments with limited money to spend, it would seem a logical option to put more money into improving people's general living conditions rather than health services, thus reducing the demand for health services in the first place.

Activity 4.10

Put yourself in the position of a government health minister. You can set up a new occupational therapy training school or refurbish a housing estate, providing insulation, central heating and leisure facilities. What would you do – you can only choose one option.

Therapists subscribing to the materialist explanation might be more inclined to get involved in and support campaigns to improve their clients' social conditions. Townsend (1993) has written very clearly about occupational therapy's social vision. She highlights that, in the development of the profession, there were elements of social and political activism, and that enabling the development of occupational potential can contribute to the promotion of social justice. She highlights occupational therapy literature that calls for therapists to advocate for social legislation and work to change the environment rather than just the individual. Townsend also makes an important point about empowering the individual in order to gain social justice.

Empowerment becomes important when we consider recent research showing that it is not just absolute poverty, but also 'relative deprivation', which is implicated in inequalities in health (Wilkinson 1997). Thus in countries such as America and the UK, even though income and standards of living may have improved, individuals still hold the same position in the overall pecking order. People may have a video and a washing machine, but they have no more power or control over their lives than they did in previous years. Thus Wilkinson suggests that it is not just the person's material well-being that is important, but also his or her position in the social hierarchy relative to others. It is in this respect – the psychosocial aspects of inequality – that therapists can help to play a role by increasing self-esteem and feelings of control.

Occupational therapy and the cultural/behavioural explanation

Therapists more inclined towards this explanation might press for more funding to get involved in health education campaigns. Because people *choose* to smoke and have a high-fat diet, the focus would be on encouraging and supporting individuals to change their unhealthy lifestyles. The intervention here is targeted on individuals and changing their behaviours. The problem with this approach is that there is little attempt to look at social forces that may be influencing individuals' behaviour. A study of 204 women in South Wales (Pill & Stott 1987) identified that they were well aware of health promotion messages about smoking and diet but, because of other social forces, stress and lack of money, did not change their behaviour. The researchers highlighted the danger of using work such as that of Lockwood discussed earlier to create stereotypes, for example those of working-class fatalism and orientation to the present.

This is, of course, not to say that attempts at health promotion and education are not useful. However, such interventions cannot alter the fact that, for example, some children live in areas where there is nowhere safe to play and are at increased risk of having an accident, or that a lifetime of manual labour can be physically damaging even with good lifting and handling skills.

CONCLUSION

From what you have read so far, it should be clear

that a concern with social class is not something restricted to Marxists: many different theorists have devised ways of classifying and identifying important differences between large groups of people in society. These distinctions have been made on the basis of occupation (Registrar-General), status (Weber) and the relationship to the means of production (Marx). Whichever scheme you adopt, it seems that there is clear evidence that the particular group to which you belong can have dramatic effects on many aspects of your life.

Given that occupational therapy is also concerned with many aspects of people's lives, it seems proper that the profession takes note of what sociologists have to say about class and stratification. If the profession is serious about having an holistic view of people, that includes taking account of the impact of social conditions and possible class-based cultural influences on individuals, their health and their beliefs about health and illness. At the same time, we need to be wary of creating stereotypes and bear in mind other influences such as gender and ethnicity.

REFERENCES

Bilton T, Bonnett K, Jones P, Stanworth M, Sheard K, Webster A 1987 Introductory sociology, 2nd edn. Macmillan, Basingstoke

Chapparo C, Ranka J 1995 Clinical reasoning in occupational therapy. In: Higgs J, Jones M (eds) Clinical reasoning in the health professions. Butterworth, London

Giddens A 1992 Sociology, 2nd edn. Polity Press, Oxford

Graham H 1987 Women's smoking and family health. Social Science and Medicine 25(1): 47–56

Haralambos M, Holborn M 1995 Sociology: themes and perspectives, 4th edn. Collins Educational, London

Hurd G, Ashton D N, Brown R K et al 1973 Human societies: an introduction to sociology. Routledge & Kegan Paul, London

Kelly G 1996 Feminist of feminine? The feminine principle in occupational therapy. British Journal of Occupational Therapy 59(1): 2–6

Krefting L H, Krefting D V 1991 Cultural influences on performance. In: Christiansen C, Baum C (eds) Occupational therapy: overcoming human performance deficits. Slack, Thorofare, NJ

Lockwood D 1966 Sources of variation in working class images of society. Cited in Haralambos M, Holborn M 1995 Sociology: themes and perspectives, 4th edn. Collins Educational, London

Mosey A C 1986 Psychosocial components of occupational therapy. Raven Press, New York

Pill R M, Stott N C H 1987 The stereotype of 'working class fatalism' and the challenge for primary care health promotion. Health Education Research 2(2): 105–114

Robinson L 1987 Patient compliance in occupational therapy home health programs: sociocultural considerations. Occupational Therapy in Health Care 4: 127–137

Scott J 1991 Who rules Britain? Polity Press, Cambridge

Times Higher Educational Supplement 1997 Rich pickings. HE success depends on postcode. April 18, no. 1276, p. 1

Townsend E 1993 Occupational therapy's social vision. Canadian Journal of Occupational Therapy 60(4): 174–183

Townsend P, Davidson N 1988 The Black Report. In: Townsend P, Davidson N, Whitehead M (eds) Inequalities in health. Penguin, Harmondsworth

US Department of Commerce 1993 Myths about elderly population dispelled by new census bureau profile of 65+ residents. US Department of Commerce News, November 10.

Westergaard J, Resler H 1976 Class in a capitalist society. Penguin, Harmondsworth

Whitehead M 1988 The health divide. In: Townsend P, Davidson N, Whitehead M (eds) Inequalities in health. Penguin, Harmondsworth

Wilkinson R G 1997 Health inequalities: relative or absolute material standards? British Medical Journal 314: 591–595

Worsley P 1977 Introducing sociology, 2nd edn. Penguin, Harmondsworth

Yelton D, Neilson C 1991 Understanding Appalachian values: implications for occupational therapists. Occupational Therapy in Mental Health 11(2/3): 173–195

5

Role

Sheena E. E. Blair

INTRODUCTION TO ROLE THEORY

The study of role and role behaviour occurs in a number of theoretical disciplines within the social sciences. Sociology is only one of those which offer a variety of theoretical views upon what constitutes the concept of role. Other disciplines that add to the body of knowledge include social anthropology, social psychology and organizational studies. It is therefore perceived as an interdisciplinary concept. In this chapter, we will explore the sociological understanding of role and role theory. This will include the emergence of the concept, theoretical positions concerning role and role behaviour, what constitutes role and its subsequent implications. Later in the chapter, we will be concerned with the importance of the concept for the practice of occupational therapy and will consider the study of role within the analysis of occupational behaviour; its theoretical integration within current models of occupational therapy and an overview of practical significance for intervention.

THE CONCEPT OF ROLE

The variety in usage of the concept of role could either add to its theoretical validity or, conversely, create some tension. Bullock et al (1988, p. 751) consider that the problem with the concept of role is its lack of restraint and pronounce that it is a 'tearaway word which tends to carry all of human behaviour indiscriminately away with it'. Despite such concerns, a consensus seems to exist that the study of role can contribute to an analysis of society and social relations. For the newcomer to any theory, attempts are usually made to seek reassurance from a definition that at least establishes a baseline for understanding. This can be found in the explanation offered by the medical sociologists Bond & Bond (1994, p. 262), who establish the importance of social context and state that 'roles are the socially defined attributes and expectations associated with social positions'. For example, in the case of a doctor (a social position), you will have certain ideas, shared by most other people, about what doctors are like and how they should behave (socially defined attributes and expectations). Thus you would expect a doctor to be well dressed, confident and, in the past, male.

Activity 5.1

Make a list of roles. You might like to start with roles relevant to yourself, for example student or sister/brother. Using the definition given by Bond & Bond (1994), add alongside your list the 'attributes and expectations' associated with the various roles you have noted.

Having gained a basic idea of the concept of role, we now need to engage in a more detailed exploration of the topic, starting with its development.

Emergence of the concept

Levin (1988) describes role, along with social structure and social status, as 'among the most basic and useful concepts' in sociology. However, investigations into the evolution of the concept of role reveal that it also originated from anthropologists, philosophers and psychologists. It is useful here briefly to review some of the key names in role theory.

Talcott Parsons

The eminent American sociologist, Parsons, had a view about role that was part of his structural functionalist perspective. He considered that

social structure could be analysed in relation to four features: values, norms, collective groups and roles. The stability of a society was, for Parsons, essentially based upon a form of harmonious order through regulation of collective activity and individual role performance. In this view, society is stable, essentially conservative and slow to change. Roles are perceived as the enactment of a preconceived part of a finely balanced society. Thus, to put it very crudely, society is composed of interdependent social institutions (the family, the workplace, universities), and within those institutions there are social positions (mother, manager, student), the people who hold those positions learning to behave in expected ways through primary or secondary socialization.

Activity 5.2

Revise your understanding of the term 'socialization'.

Robert K. Merton

Merton (1957) was also a sociologist in the functionalist tradition, modifying some of the original Parsonian ideas and, within the context of role theory, being responsible for the origin of the term 'role-set'. This describes the range and complexity of expectations surrounding any one individual who carries out a role. We will explore this concept in more detail later on. Although Merton is regarded as a functionalist, his approach to role indicates a degree of flexibility. He believed that control is exerted over behaviour:

- through clearly defined rules or laws specifying what one must do
- through less clearly defined expectations held by oneself and others regarding what one ought to do
- through habit, custom and routine.

This seems to suggest a synthesis between the functionalists and those interested in the meanings that individuals attach to situations (the interpretavists). Thus Merton refers to laws (a structural feature) but also allows for some flexibility through recognition of the existence of ill-defined expectations.

George Herbert Mead

A different notion of role emerged from the work of Mead, a social philosopher who was influential in the development of symbolic interactionism. You will remember from Chapter 2 that symbolic interactionism falls within the sociological perspective sometimes broadly referred to as interpretavist. In sociological terms, this is known as a micro-level theory because it is concerned with more intimate face-to-face interaction rather than with social institutions. The essence of this theory is that interaction is a learned social process, which, according to Goodman (1992), 'occurs through symbols or representations that have agreed meanings'. It relies on the belief that people interpret interactions and reactions, and imagine themselves in another's position. This infers that the enacting of roles is dynamic: they are constantly being reinterpreted and are open to negotiation.

R. H. Turner and Harold Garfinkel

Turner (1962) was a theorist in the tradition of Mead and was responsible for objecting to the idea, from the structural functionalist tradition, of 'role-taking', which inferred that all roles were prescribed and regulated by rules. He suggested an alternative – 'role-making' – which involved negotiation and the individual interpretation of situations.

Garfinkel (1967) is another theorist within this tradition. He worked on concepts that were designed to impose caution on the idea of an ordered social world. Garfinkel is particularly associated with ethnomethodology, a perspective that, according to the definition given by Goodman (1992), directs attention to how people view order in the world, how they communicate that view to others and how they understand and explain social interaction. Thus the study of role within this frame of reference is again concerned with perceptions and consequent actions.

Criticisms exist of the interpretavist and func-

tionalist perspectives. More micro-level theories in the tradition of Mead are considered to negate the importance of formal organizational aspects of society. On the other hand, macro-level theories, in particular structural functionalism, are considered to be too simplistic an explanation for the complexity of modern life and the interactions occurring within it.

Activity 5.3

At this point in the development of your knowledge about role theory, are you attracted to the view that we put on roles, like an overcoat, depending on our social position at any specific time? Or do you prefer the idea that roles, and therefore attributes and expectations, are negotiated?

Consider professions or jobs that seem to have more opportunity or licence for interpretation of roles. For example, contrast the roles of a soldier and a student.

FUNCTIONALIST AND INTERACTIONIST PERSPECTIVES ON ROLE

The two main perspectives on role have, through the work of particular theorists such as Parsons and Mead, already been introduced and will now be explored in more detail.

Functionalism

Functionalism, which was the dominant perspective in sociology in the mid-twentieth century, maintains that relationships between members of a society are organized in terms of rules in a network of interacting systems. Stable expectations and behaviours are developed through the role relationships that arise. In turn, these expectations enable others to meet them and to carry out role obligations in return for the rights that are attached to their respective roles. Behaviour is therefore made predictable, and society persists even though its members change. One of the functions of socialization is to prepare the individual for different roles in the social system.

The occupier of a role, or the role incumbent,

as Bond & Bond (1994) describes it must show appropriate feelings and values. In this respect, according to functionalist views, the family in particular is regarded as vital to the social structure, in that it plays a vital part in passing on appropriate role behaviours. Parsons (1964) provides the fullest account of the family in teaching, for example, gender roles within primary socialization. The learning of more complex social rules in later childhood and adulthood takes place during secondary socialization.

One of the problems with functionalism is that it has difficulty explaining social change. If everything is interdependent, i.e. if things are organized in a certain way because it helps society to work, and people learn how to behave in expected ways from an early age, how and why do societies change? We can restate this point in sociological language and say that one of the main criticisms of functionalism is its essential conservatism, which fails to give an adequate explanation for social change, so subsequently maintains the *status quo*.

Symbolic interactionism

Symbolic interactionism, in contrast to functionalism, is more concerned with how an individual comes to be defined in a certain way. While functionalists imply that roles are provided by the social system, and the individual enacts his role as if reading from a script, interactionists argue that roles are less clear, often being ambiguous and vague. This lack of clarity allows room for negotiation, roles, at best, offering general guidelines for action. This is a more dynamic view of role behaviour, which is seen to occur within an interaction process. As Haralambos & Holborn (1990) state, while interactionists admit the existence of roles, they regard them as vague and therefore open to negotiation and change. One of the most famous sociologists from the interactionist school is Erving Goffman.

Erving Goffman

Another account of roles can be read in Goffman (1987), who puts the notion of role into the idea of types and believes that the construction of role types is a necessary aspect of the institutionalization of conduct. All roles represent institutional order, but some are of more strategic importance to society. Historically, roles representing institutional order have been located in political and religious institutions. Goffman reiterates, however, that learning a role, as functionalists seem to suggest, is not sufficient. He argues that one must be initiated into various cognitive and affective layers of the body of knowledge that is directly and indirectly appropriate to the role. For example, a student may have discovered that learning to become a therapist and the inculcation of professional attitudes is a complex and varied process.

The other aspect of Goffman's work for which he is well known is his use of a 'dramaturgical model'. This term is used to emphasize the, often deliberate, way in which people 'play' with roles like actors interpreting or improvising with a script. In the *Presentation of self in everyday life* (Goffman 1971), he describes how waiters, for example, play out their role to an almost exaggerated degree when 'on show' in the public areas of a restaurant, only to let this front relax when in the kitchen. In fact, behaviour in what Goffman calls the 'backstage areas' of role performance can be the reverse of public behaviour. For example, the waiter polite and respectful to customers while serving can turn into the opposite as soon as he enters the kitchen, swearing and making rude comments about the same people.

Activity 5.4

Can you think of instances in which you have observed therapists 'playing' at their role in the way Goffman suggests?

How does therapists' behaviour in the 'backstage' area of the staff room differ from their 'on-stage' performance? What would happen if a client inadvertently entered this backstage area?

Goffman's work fits very well with the notion that we do not simply take on roles but that we manipulate and develop them. That is to say, we make roles.

Role-taking and role-making

Any social position may require some negotiation. Some sociologists have emphasized the important distinction between role-taking and role-making. The idea of role-taking suggests that all roles are prescribed and defined by a specific set of rules to which everyone will conform, for example soldiers in the army or traffic wardens. Bond & Bond (1994) state they do as 'the system' prescribes; thus this fits in with a functionalist perspective. Alternatively, the idea of role-making suggests that roles are created, moulded and modified by individuals themselves, according to their own interpretation, and is therefore more in concert with an interactionist perspective.

CONCEPTS ASSOCIATED WITH ROLE THEORY

We have seen that the idea of role is a complex one and subject to many different approaches. From the brief overview of theoretical positions concerning role, it is clear that it is a dynamic concept. Leaving aside this debate, it is useful to consider some of the other important concepts associated with role theory.

Role and status

As we have seen, some authors believe role to be a useful concept because it helps to define and analyse some forms of social interaction, i.e. what is going on when two people meet. The concept of status is also useful as it gives an indication of the position of a particular role in a social hierarchy. Levin (1988) makes the following distinction between status and role:

- *Social status*: a position or place within a social structure to which certain rights and obligations apply. For example, professional status offers the individual an elevated place in society, with attendant rewards and privileges.
- *Social role*: the behaviour expected of an individual because of the social status

occupied. For example, the behaviour expected of a health professional is specific expertise and proven ability to alter the illness or problem experienced by an individual.

In practice, the term 'role' is often used to describe both the position and the behaviour. Linton (1936), an anthropologist, differentiated between:

- *ascribed status*, which is the aspects over which you have no control, i.e. being born a son or daughter, male or female
- *achieved status*, resulting from something the individual has done, for example attaining a particular occupational position.

Some authors, for example Oatley (1990), have considered that the idea of roles and the associated concept of status are problematic in modern societies. Roles and status are now more fluid; there is much more likely to be debate over the status of a particular role now compared with earlier in the twentieth century. While changes within society have required a re-examination of the concept of roles and status, they nevertheless continue to act as useful units of analysis of social behaviour. For example, the status of professionals has, it could be argued, changed, although their role has not – or not to the same extent, or in the same way. Another feature of modern societies is the way in which people juggle multiple roles.

Multiple roles

The pace of life in industrialized societies at the end of the twentieth century involves people undertaking many different roles at any one particular time of life. An example is given in Figure 5.1. The picture becomes more complex when we consider that each of these roles interconnects with a set of complementary roles.

Activity 5.5

At this point, consider yourself for a few minutes and note *all* the roles that you fulfil within the course of a day.

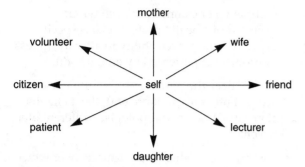

Figure 5.1 Multiple roles.

Role-set

Merton (1957) used the term 'role-set' to describe the network of relationships that surrounds a particular role. Figure 5.2 gives an indication of the possible role-set of a lecturer. Of course, not all the roles in a set have equal influence or importance. For example, the relationship between the lecturer and head of department will be more important than that between the lecturer and the canteen staff.

The complexity of people's lives becomes clear when we begin to attach the role-sets to the multiple roles that individuals hold. There is a clear difference between the role and role-set that is experienced as a mother and as a lecturer. Thus the potential for conflict between roles is high.

Role conflict

As social life has become increasingly complex and competitive, the incidence of conflict, or

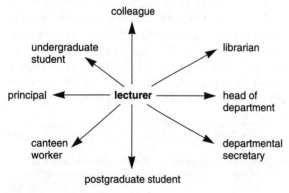

Figure 5.2 Role-set.

strain, increases. The more roles one holds, the greater the possibility of conflict between them, and the larger one's role-set, the greater the possibility of competing expectations. Conflict may be experienced as a result of:

- conflict from incompatible expectations, for example a proposal for team-building initiatives after hours or at weekends producing conflict between the role of co-worker and member of the family
- overload arising from demands beyond the worker's capacity, for example conflict between the demand for research and a high quality of teaching
- ambiguity, for example when there is a lack of clear information about what is expected of a worker and uncertainly about the outcome of work and job performance.

Various studies suggest that the greater the diversity of a role-set, the greater the chance of a conflict within a role. The interaction of multiple roles has been written about by Runciman (1982) from a nursing perspective. She discovered that the role-set of the ward sister consists of over 100 role relationships, suggesting it to be no surprise that the nurse feels required to meet everyone's expectations and that these expectations are not always met.

> **Activity 5.6**
>
> As a result of becoming a student, have you experienced role conflict?

Role loss and transition

Whether you subscribe to the functionalist or interactionist conception of roles, there is no doubt that the disruption of those roles through illness or other life events (retirement, death of a partner or children leaving home) has major consequences for an individual. This is because roles provide a major source of identity regardless of whether we make or take them. When we describe ourselves, it is usually in terms of the roles we undertake – daughter, mother, lecturer, friend, etc. – and the loss of any of these roles requires readjustment. The threat to personal equilibrium is greater if a number of roles are lost simultaneously, but the loss of any valued role will create a vacuum and require adaptive responses.

Role transitions

The adaptation to various role transitions involves relinquishing valued role positions, seen for example in the change required in parental roles as children leave home or in the reconstruction of the self that is required after a painful separation or divorce. In this respect, there are few 'scripts' available, and the individual is in an unfamiliar position in which old habits and routines are redundant and a new identity needs to be constructed.

It is the engagement in roles and the emotional overlay that has interested Oatley (1990). His belief is that 'although emotions can effect role transactions, and emotions can result from role transactions, they can also themselves be transitional roles'. Emotions may function to readjust roles that have become unsatisfactory or stagnant. They may provide the momentum for change in either the redefinition or the termination of a role.

Roles and health

The loss of role and the adaptation to new roles is very much tied up with health issues. Becoming ill may result in the loss of the role of worker. Someone else becoming ill or dying may result in the loss of the role of daughter/son, or a person may have to give up one role in order to undertake another, for example that of carer. One of the key concepts in relation to roles and health comes from Parsons, who developed the notion of the sick role.

Sick role

This has become an overused and often pejorative description of the perceived dependent behaviour of people who have difficulty func-

tioning within society. However, if used with care, it can highlight the nature of interactions between a person defined as 'sick' and those with whom they interact.

The idea was developed by Parsons (1951), who outlined the nature of the expectations surrounding illness, which he regarded as a form of deviance. You will remember that for Parsons, as a functionalist, a key concern was the identification of the means by which social order is maintained. Illness is regarded as a form of deviance as it poses a threat to that social order because the individual is no longer able to perform his or her expected roles. To deal with this situation, there are people who perform the role of doctor and are expected to identify and treat people who become patients, i.e. take on the sick role. The behaviour of the sick person and that of those in a position to care all conform to a certain pattern of role expectations.

You will remember how, earlier in this chapter, we talked about some of the attributes and expectations surrounding the role of doctor; similarly, Parsons has identified a number of key features of the sick role (Box 5.1). Using the concept of role-set, we can begin to see the network of relationships – the role-set – surrounding the person who is ill.

Criticisms of the sick role

Despite the popularity of the concept of the sick role among health professionals, it is not without its critics. A broad criticism is that,

---

Box 5.1 Key features of the sick role

- People in the sick role can legitimately claim exemption from normal activities and responsibilities
- The status of being sick affords assistance and the right to be dependent upon others

However, there are certain obligations associated with this role, including:

- the wish to get well and relinquish the sick role as soon as possible
- the requirement to recover by acting in the appropriate manner, for example by taking medicine

---

like functionalism generally, it is concerned with normality and the maintenance of order. One big issue is that of the power of the medical and associated professions to define exactly who is ill and therefore has a valid claim to the sick role. It is interesting to note the problems that people with chronic pain or chronic fatigue syndrome often have in terms of being labelled as malingerers because doctors can find no identifiable pathology. Another problem highlighted by this example is that while Parsons' concept might have some validity in relation to acute illness, it is not easily applicable to chronic illness yet it is often used in this way.

Activity 5.7

In a small group, discuss situations in which therapists with whom you have been in contact have used the concept of the sick role. How valid was the use of the concept, and was it the only explanation of an individual's behaviour?

Make a list of conditions in which individuals' claims to being considered ill might be rejected.

ROLE THEORY AND THE PRACTICE OF OCCUPATIONAL THERAPY

A profession that is based upon understanding the occupational nature of human beings is bound to be concerned with the nature and meaning of role behaviour. According to a position statement regarding core skills by the British College of Occupational Therapy (1994), occupational therapy has, since its inception, sought to contribute to health through 'the use of activities, occupations, skills and life roles which enable people to function purposefully in their daily life'. However, the notion of role is often uncritically dealt with in occupational therapy literature and supposes a theoretical 'given'. Many articles claim to explore and outline the 'role' of occupational therapy in a particular area without any examination of the concept. A sociological understanding of role permits a more thorough analysis of the influences that impinge upon behaviour and fosters an understanding of the social construction of professional roles. More specifically it:

- assists therapists to be more informed about role behaviour in all aspects of intervention
- enables therapists to locate core skills within various theoretical approaches concerning role
- facilitates an understanding of the context in which people adopt and sustain various roles.

This part of the chapter will examine these issues and the theoretical importance of the concept of role for current models of occupational therapy.

Activity 5.8

Before continuing with this chapter, go to the library and, from browsing catalogues or a CD ROM search, identify articles written in occupational therapy journals concerned with the role of the occupational therapist in any particular area.

ROLE-TAKING AND ROLE-MAKING IN OCCUPATIONAL THERAPY

We saw earlier in this chapter how it is possible to view roles as being adopted in a very mechanistic way or alternatively being negotiated within a broad framework. It is often implied in journal articles and elsewhere that the role of the therapist is absolute, clear cut and unquestionable. Thus one may detect a functionalist perspective suggesting that role-taking can be identified. Within the first block of fieldwork practice, occupational therapy students are often asked briefly to explore the role of occupational therapy in that area. This typically produces a description and list of the activities carried out by the therapist. However, with more reflection, the student and supervisor may begin to examine a number of factors. Upon further reading, one may come across work, for example Robinson (1984), in which it becomes evident that therapists have negotiated their position very astutely and are therefore engaged in role-making.

The manner in which the role of the occupational therapist is constructed and whether it is prescribed in formal ways or is negotiated within a team may be dictated by the setting.

In this respect, discrepancies may be noted, as in the experience of Fairhurst (1981), in which the official occupational ideology proposed by the organization in which she worked was not shared by practising occupational therapists. Here, therapists negotiated their own identity through the skilful perception of social forces and succeeded in establishing a revised role.

Activity 5.9

Read again the explanation of 'role-taking' and 'role-making' and consider what was evident in your most recent fieldwork experience.

Role conflict

Where we find negotiation of role, it should come as no surprise that there are more opportunities for role conflict. It can be useful to explore the issue of role strain or conflict within various settings. The clearest example of this may be within community and mental health settings where work had previously been carried out within the context of an institution. Negotiation of new realities concerning role boundaries is a daily occurrence and can cause tensions as people may try to recreate the rigid roles that belong in other contexts. Efforts consciously to develop interdisciplinary teamwork can be seen as an attempt to reduce role conflict.

From the examination so far of role in relation to occupational therapy, one would expect to find the concept given a high profile and critical examination within the literature, but this is not necessarily the case.

ROLE IN OCCUPATIONAL THERAPY LITERATURE

While all occupational therapists will, in the course of their work, consider the habitual roles of their clients (as spouse, parent or worker) and, in theory, the meanings embedded within those roles, the frank acknowledgement of role as a key concept in practice has, at least in British texts, been more implicit than explicit.

A key book such as Creek's (1996) on occu-pational therapy in mental health includes a chapter on roles and settings, but this contains no critical analysis of the theoretical underpinning. It does, however, consider important issues such as balancing roles and problems with role iden-tification. Others, notably Hagedorn (1992) and Young & Quinn (1992), refer to role only in terms of the position held by the concept of role within the model of human occupation (MOHO). This omission is interesting considering the number of times the literature on occupational therapy heralds the uniqueness of the role of the occu-pational therapist in a plethora of settings.

Role in American literature

In the American literature, the centrality of the concept of role for the process of occupational therapy is more apparent within occupational therapy models of practice, but only Matsutsuyu (1971) attempts to place role and role behaviour within a sociological context. She considers that the occupational behaviour frame of reference is partly based upon the sociological concept of role and socialization. Reed & Sanderson (1992) also deal with the concept of role within an ex-planation of role behaviour in which the steady acquisition of skills increases the individual's ability to adapt. Examples are given of role development and possibilities for intervention by occupational therapists to enhance abilities and facilitate synthesis between individual need and social expectation. It is within the well-known model of human occupation (Kielhofner 1985, 1992), however, that an acknowledgement of the importance of roles for the practice of occupational therapy is a key feature.

Role and MOHO

This approach to conceptualizing the focus of occupational therapy is constantly being researched with all client groups and has gained support on both sides of the Atlantic. The model evolved from the pioneering work of Reilly (1962), who emphasized the need to study and research occupations in a specific way for the advancement of the profession. MOHO views

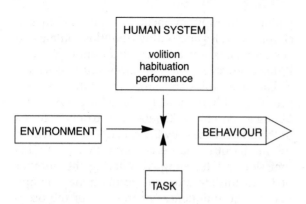

Figure 5.3 Behaviour results from an interaction between the human system, the environment and the task (adapted with permission from Kielhofner & Forsyth 1997).

the human being as an open system comprising three subsystems (Fig. 5.3). This is explained by Kielhofner (1992, p. 166) as a 'composition of interrelated structures and functions organised into a coherent whole that interacts with an environment and is capable of maintaining and changing itself'. The subsystems exist in a heterarchy, the entire system being interrelated and transactional.

The volitional subsystem is concerned with the person's sense of effectiveness and control. It also includes a value system that determines whether or not a person will become involved in an occupation. Finally, it contains a component on interests and preferences based upon range, pattern and balance of involvement in those occupations.

It is within the habituation subsystem, which is responsible for organizing behaviours into routines, that the notion of role assumes an important position. In the definition by Kielhofner (1992, p. 158), roles 'are images that persons hold about the positions they occupy in various social groups and of the obligations that go along with those positions'. Role balance is an important element within MOHO and, as the term

---

Activity 5.10

Examine this definition carefully and consider which sociological theory concerning role it resembles.

---

suggests, is concerned with the degree to which the individual satisfactorily integrates roles with a daily pattern of living.

The final subsystem – the performance subsystem – is one that allows the individual to carry out tasks, processes and interactions with others. Three types of skill are contained within this subsystem:

- perceptual-motor skills
- process skills, such as cognitive abilities
- communication/interaction skills.

This is an important model for the practice of occupational therapy, through which the assessment of an individual can appraise whether an adaptive or maladaptive cycle is apparent. In terms of role behaviour, it is adaptive if balance, enjoyment and challenge are experienced, but maladaptive if role loss, imbalance or strain reinforces a feeling of uselessness. Within this dynamic system, as Hagedorn (1992) notes, changes in any part of the whole system reverberate throughout the entire experience of an individual. A key argument of the model is that different parts of the human system can adapt to alteration within another, thereby restoring balance. The job of the occupational therapist is to help the individual in this process. The model has produced a number of assessments to analyse human behaviour, including a role checklist providing information on roles, habits, interests and routines. Other assessment tools include the Occupational Case Analysis Interview and Rating Scale (OCAIRS) (Kaplan & Kielhofner 1989), which includes an important section on perceived roles. In terms of role behaviour, this model ascertains that disorder and problems occur for the individual where loss of role results in the disorganization of behaviour.

Functionalist bias within MOHO

There are clearly many parallels between MOHO and the sociological literature on role. It is also possible to detect that there is generally a more functionalist than interactionist ethos apparent in the model. One obvious link is the fact that, like the work of the functionalist Talcott Parsons,

MOHO is based on systems theory. Earlier, you were asked to examine Kielhofner's definition of role, and you no doubt identified that, with its focus on 'obligations', it suggests a more rigid conception of role. Elsewhere, Kielhofner & Forsyth (1997, p. 107) note, 'The concept of role argues that people perform within positions in a social group, exhibiting patterns of interaction, task performance and time use that reflect expectations associated with the role.' Once again, this is more suggestive of role-taking than role-making.

In contrast, Hillman and Chapparo (1995), writing from an Australian perspective, emphasize the fact that the same person may view the same activity, and therefore its attachment to a particular role, as being different in different circumstances.

Role in Australian literature

Chapparo has been connected with research, ongoing since the mid-1980s, concerning a model of occupational role performance. Within this model, occupational role is defined as 'patterns of behaviour composed of self maintenance, work, leisure and rest activities' (Hillman & Chapparo 1995). Occupational role performance – the way in which these activities are carried out – is defined as 'the means by which people express themselves, achieve an identity within their own society and find meaning in their lives'

(Hillman & Chapparo 1997, p. 405). Notice how the association here is between role and activity, with less emphasis on attributions and expectations, which seem to be highlighted in the sociological literature. This model can be represented diagrammatically (Fig. 5.4).

The degree to which this model explains the interaction between individuals and their context is of interest. The model also acknowledges the understanding of the individuality of people and how that becomes evident in subsequent role performance. They note that 'In describing role performance, health professionals often make assumptions about the meaning and balance that is ascribed by clients to their own life roles' (Hillman & Chapparo 1995, p. 89). However, it is also interesting to compare the diagrammatic representations of MOHO and the model of occupational role performance. Note how the latter also seems to imply a systems approach, with its three elements resulting in occupational role performance, and how satisfaction operates as a feedback mechanism that re-enters the loop.

Examination of both the American and Australian literature highlights the importance of having a clear understanding of the way in which the term 'role' is being used and recognizing that there are different perspectives on the concept. The complexity of the issue can be seen by the fact that Kielhofner's work can at times sound very functionalist, while at the same time,

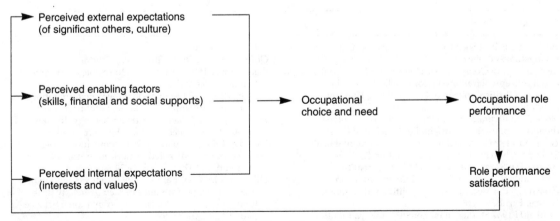

Figure 5.4 Model of occupational role performance (From Hillman & Chapparo 1995 with permission, adapted from Heard 1977)

in other places, he emphasizes the importance of the individual's experience, utilizing the work of Turner and other interactionists (Kielhofner & Forsyth 1997). In the same way, Chapparo's work emphasizes individual experience but, when represented diagrammatically, looks very much like a systems model. Whichever model one adopts, it is important to be aware of the danger of role-stereotyping.

ROLE-STEREOTYPING

Any model that views role as given rather than made is in danger of reinforcing stereotyped views of what a particular role entails and fails to recognize cultural differences in role expectations. Thus certain activities become 'role-bound'; for example, home maintenance might typically be considered to be part of the male role.

The problem of stereotypical roles and the way in which they might influence the choice of an activity within therapy is an important consideration. Tasks and activities can be invested with assumptions that are powerful and disempowering. This may be evident in activities that have a strong gender bias or age-linked bias. Treatment programmes often reflect what is deemed to be age appropriate, but there are, of course, notable exceptions. In the uncritical choice of bingo for older people or kitchen activities for women, strong role-type prejudice can be detected.

Activity 5.11
Consider experiences from fieldwork and note activities that seemed 'role-bound'.

CONCLUSION

In conclusion, the study of occupational performance is incomplete without the inclusion of an analysis of role. It is intrinsically bound up with identity and the presentation of self in an increasingly complex world. We have seen how we can use sociological concepts such as role-taking and role-making to analyse the role of the occupational therapist and his or her control over it; we have also shown how the concept of role-set can be used to identify the complex web of relationships in which therapists are engaged. An examination of the concept of the sick role has shown that we need to be aware of the complexity and limitations of these ideas, and we have identified how the occupational therapy literature sometimes fails to acknowledge the complexity surrounding the notion of role. After reading this chapter, you should now be in a better position to evaluate work in occupational therapy on role.

REFERENCES

Bond J, Bond S 1994 Sociology and health care. Churchill Livingstone, Edinburgh

British College of Occupational Therapy 1994 Core skills and a conceptual framework for practice: a position statement. British College of Occupational Therapy, London

Bullock A, Stallybrass O, Trombley S 1988 The Fontana dictionary of modern thought. Fontana Press, Glasgow

Creek J (ed.) 1996 Occupational therapy and mental health 2nd edn. Churchill Livingstone, Edinburgh

Fairhurst E 1981 What do you do? Multiple realities in occupational therapy rehabilitation. In: Aitkinson P, Hoach C (eds) Medical work – realities and routines. Gower, Farnborough

Garfinkel H 1967 Studies in ethnomethodology. Prentice Hall, Englewood Cliffs, NJ

Goffman E 1971 The presentation of self in everyday life. Pelican, London

Goffman E 1987 Roles. Tavistock, London

Goodman N 1992 Introduction to sociology. Harper Perennial, New York

Hagedorn R 1992 Occupational therapy: foundations for practice. Churchill Livingstone, Edinburgh

Haralambos M, Holborn M 1990 Sociology: themes and perspectives, 3rd edn. Unwin Hyman, London

Heard C 1977 Occupational role acquisition: a perspective on the chronically disabled. American Journal of Occupational Therapy 31(4): 243–247

Hillman A M, Chapparo C J 1995 An investigation of occupational performance in men over sixty years of age, following a stroke. Journal of Occupational Science (Australia) 2(3): 88–99

Kaplan K L, Kielhofner G 1989 Occupational case analysis interview and rating scale. Slack, Thorofare, NJ

Kielhofner G 1985 A model of human occupation. Williams & Wilkins, Baltimore, MD

Kielhofner G 1992 Conceptual foundations of occupational therapy. F. A. Davis, Philadelphia

Kielhofner G, Forsyth K 1997 The model of human occupation: an overview of current concepts. British Journal of Occupational Therapy 60(3): 103–110

Levin W C 1988 Sociological ideas, concepts and applications. Wadsworth, Belmont, CA

Linton R 1936 The study of man. Appleton-Century-Crofts, New York

Matsutsuyu J 1971 Occupational behaviour – a perspective on work and play. American Journal of Occupational Therapy XXV(6): 291–294

Merton R K 1957 The role-set: problems in sociological theory. British Journal of Sociology 8: 106–120

Oatley K 1990 Role transitions and the emotional structure of everyday life. In Fisher S & Cooper C L (eds) On the move – the psychology of change and transition. John Wiley, Chichester

Parsons T 1951 The social system. Routledge & Kegan Paul, London

Parsons T 1964 Social structure and personality. Free Press, New York

Reed K L, Sanderson S N 1992 Concepts of occupational therapy. Williams & Wilkins, Baltimore, MD

Reilly M 1962 Occupational therapy can be one of the great ideas of 20th century medicine. American Journal of Occupational Therapy 16: 1

Robinson E 1984 The role of the occupational therapist in a psychotherapeutic setting. British Journal of Occupational Therapy 47(4)

Runciman P 1982 Ward sisters: their problems at work – 2. Nursing Times Occasional Paper 78(51): 145–147

Turner R H 1962 Role-taking: process versus conforming. In: Rose A M (ed.) Human behaviour and social processes. Routledge & Kegan Paul, London

Young M E, Quinn E 1992 Theories and principles of occupational therapy. Churchill Livingstone, Edinburgh

FURTHER READING

Berger P L 1975 Invitation to sociology. Pelican, Harmondsworth

Berger P, Luckmann T 1987. The social construction of reality. Penguin, Harmondsworth

6

Sex, gender and feminism

Doreen MacWhannell

Sheena E. E. Blair

QUESTIONS OF SEX AND GENDER

Occupational therapy is a predominantly female profession (Miller 1992). It is also defined as one of the 'helping' or 'caring' professions. These facts raise interesting questions for the women and men who might come into contact with occupational therapists and for therapists themselves. At the same time, discussion of the nature of caring work may lead to the conclusion that it is commonly defined as 'women's work'. Consideration of these questions highlights the importance of issues of sex and gender for health-care professions such as occupational therapy.

This chapter will begin by considering the terms 'sex' and 'gender', and their position within sociological theory. Use of the terms 'feminine'/ 'femininity' and 'masculine'/'masculinity' is considered in order to allow an understanding of what they mean in relation to sex and gender. This chapter will therefore seek to:

- define female and male in relation to sex and gender
- define the concept of social construction in order to understand femininity and masculinity
- address the concept of sex/gender role-stereotyping
- consider the influence of feminist perspectives on sociological thought
- relate feminist perspectives to occupational therapy practice.

UNTANGLING SEX AND GENDER

A key issue in the sociological literature is the distinction that is made between sex and gender. It should be noted that, although sociologists tend to make clear distinctions between sex and gender, the terms are often used interchangeably in everyday life *and* in some of the literature.

The biology of sex

> **Activity 6.1**
>
> Can you define your sex?

A common approach to explaining what sex is is to begin by studying sex *differences*, i.e. what distinguishes females from males. Discussing these differences often leads to listing anatomical or physiological features. For example, females have ovaries, fallopian tubes, a cervix and a vagina; males have a penis, prostate and testicles. These are physical features, not all of which are visible. Further discussion can lead to noting other biological features – chromosomal and hormonal differences.

> **Activity 6.2**
>
> List other biological and physical differences between the sexes.

Biological differences such as the fact that women menstruate and may bear children might appear in your list from Activity 6.2. Interestingly, even the initial, apparently clear, biological basis of inquiry has its complications. For example, the hormone testosterone, which is often thought of as being a 'male' hormone, is found in both men and women. The difference lies in the levels in which it is present.

You may also have included in your list differences in physical characteristics such as height, weight and skeletal and muscular development. This latter list is more problematic as such a *variety* of differences exist between and among women and men. Oakley (1985) reminds us that sexual differences vary between and within ethnic

groups. For example, most people probably think of males as being taller than females, but would this be the case if we compared the heights of Norwegian females and Japanese males? Even within an ethnic group, some females will be bigger and stronger than some males – think of women body-builders. Although clear anatomical differences are present between most females and males, each person can be considered to be an individual existing somewhere along a continuum in terms of height, hormone levels, etc.

Biology and behaviour

Some researchers believe that biological sex differences are essentially responsible for determining the social roles of women and men. As Stacey (1993, p. 68) puts it, 'essentialism refers to arguments which appeal to biological or genetic determinism, universalism or explanations based on the idea of "nature" or "human nature"'. This applies to sociologists (hence the term sociobiology), psychologists and anthropologists as well as physiologists and biologists. The debate around the role of biology in determining behaviour is controversial, and, as we shall see later in this chapter, other researchers and theorists adopt a stance in which culture rather than biology is seen to inform social roles and behaviour.

The importance of language to this discussion must be noted. The aforementioned discussion on difference resulting from biology encourages us to consider a continuum with 'female', as a sex, at one end, and 'male', as a sex, at the other. Despite this continuum, the terms 'woman' and 'man' are applied to individuals, i.e. they are allocated to one category or the other.

Difficulties arise when considering other differences between women and men, especially when these are neither biological, physical nor physiological. The discussion is complicated when attempts are made to discuss attributes and characteristics and to ascribe these to women and men. For example, it is commonly believed that women will develop feminine traits and men masculine traits. This leads us on to the consideration of the term 'gender'.

Gender

Oakley (1985 p. 158) notes that 'Sex is a biological term; 'gender' is a psychological and cultural one.' In other words, the female sex, for example, need not automatically belong to the corresponding (feminine) gender, and therefore being a woman or a man is as much a function of dress, gesture, occupation, social network and personality as it is of possessing a certain set of genitals.

A more useful way to think about this is to consider an individual's degree of femininity and/or masculinity. The mix or degree of gender found in an individual is an interesting concept. Some would consider it controversial to consider that there are 'degrees' of femininity and or 'masculinity' in all of us. It may be questioned whether such universal categorizing can be applied.

Femininity and masculinity

Activity 6.3
Try to define 'feminine' and 'masculine'.

In attempting to debate a statement such as 'Women are more feminine than men', we are challenged into defining norms and normality, i.e. 'normal' for a woman or 'normal' for a man. Clear differences are often cited and polarized around whether women or men possess certain attributes, qualities or characteristics. Consider the adjective 'aggressive' and ask yourself to which sex this word is most commonly attributed. As Oakley (1985) notes, 'aggression has become a key word in the literature on sex differences and is used to cover a considerable range of behaviours and temperamental traits'. Aggression is commonly constructed in the literature as a masculine (male) 'trait', but Oakley (1985) challenges this assumption by arguing that the differences between girls and boys in aggression are not 'absolute' but 'latent'. She demonstrates this by referring to research in this area stating that girls use verbal aggression more than boys, and boys use physical aggression more than girls. Within her text, she clearly demonstrates

that traits attributed to one sex or another can be challenged and contested by other researchers and have much to do with social rules and the ways in which girls and boys, and women and men, are socialized into particular societies.

The debate here has started to shift from one of biological sex differences that determine whether we are described as women or men to something else concerning differences that appear to be more fluid, less exact and able to shift. At this point, it is necessary to discuss the social construction of sex and gender.

SOCIAL CONSTRUCTION OF SEX AND GENDER

It is important here to return to Oakley's definition of gender being a psychological and cultural term; it is the latter that will be addressed. The question of how we become women and men is a far more complicated debate than that of 'biology', where being born with a particular set of genitals determines, for example, whether the girl baby grows to be a woman. Social constructionism appeals to the idea that these categories are not natural, fixed or universal but specific to the social, cultural and historical context. Consider the following statements from de Beauvoir (1976):

Woman? Very simple, say the fanciers of simple formulas: she is a womb, an ovary; she is female ...

One is not born, but rather becomes, a woman.

It is the word 'becomes' that is useful in offering us a way in which to understand the concept of gender. It also allows us to move beyond the constraints of what were at first thought to be clearly defined and fixed categories of woman and man.

Social constructionism would particularly challenge biological explanations for the roles that women and men typically play within society. It is helpful to consider the role of motherhood in this context. While women are physically able to bear a child, this does not mean that all women would wish to bear a child and assume the role of mother. This raises questions such as:

- Is motherhood 'natural' for women?

- Is 'caring' a more 'natural' role for women than men?
- Is 'fatherhood' a natural role for men?

That gender identity can be seen to be socially constructed according to the particular society one lives in is illustrated by the following example. On the birth of a baby, identification of her genitals determines that she is of the female sex. She is defined as a baby girl. The midwives in the maternity unit identify her cot and wrist with name tags that are coloured pink.

Activity 6.4

Why is the colour 'pink' used? Why does this practice occur? What does it mean to take such action?

The colour pink has been socially constructed as belonging to girls and women, i.e. those who are defined as female. This is a tradition within Western society and is based on custom and practice. Blue is constructed as a 'male' (masculine) colour. The use of colour has been used here to highlight and identify common constructions of everyday events that can traditionally begin to take on more meaning than was intended. Modern society can challenge such constructs; for example, in today's fashion industry 'anything goes', but there was once a time when it was considered unusual for a man to wear pink – the man was wearing a 'feminine' colour. Children's toys today still demonstrate common notions of femininity and masculinity: think of Barbie and Action Man!

This simple example has been used to demonstrate the origins of how social constructions of femininity and masculinity can be used. In this instance, we can see attempts to fix clear categories of difference when this is not in fact possible. It was stated above that gender is a more fluid, less fixed and static category than a biological construct. Yet the examples above have demonstrated how attempts are made to fix constructions of gender and ascribe polarized gender constructs. It is suggested here that this is neither useful nor constructive to both women and men.

Activity 6.5

List other examples of where attempts are made to ascribe fixed gendered categories. Consider the following list and think back to your early childhood. How did the fact that you were ascribed a specific gender affect:

- your clothes
- how you spoke
- the books you were given
- the toys you were given
- your activities at school
- your activities at play?

Levin (1988) noted that, by the age of 3, American children have an idea about what are the 'correct' activities for girls and boys and the types of job that men and women do. Having seen how our ideas about male and female, masculine and feminine, are socially constructed, we can now look at the way in which social roles are allocated to one or other category.

SEX/GENDERED ROLES

We have seen that an individual is ascribed both a sex and a gender. The question to be raised here is whether this ascribed gender determines the roles assumed and played out in adult life, for example in work, and within and outside the home. Chapter 5 has dealt with role theories, but it would be useful at this point to consider sex role-stereotyping within the discussion. This can be understood as the ascribing of fixed expectations about the social positions attributed to men and women. Eitzen (1980, p. 154) notes that, before the 1960s, American women were expected to be 'passive, submissive, gentle, dependent, family orientated, emotional, sentimental, idealistic and intuitive.' Of course, things have changed since then – or have they?

Activity 6.6

Consider the following list. How does the fact that you are ascribed a specific sex or gender affect:

- the jobs you have had
- your behaviour as a single or married man/woman
- what domestic tasks you do or are expected to do
- your leisure choices?

One question to be raised here concerns the choice to become an occupational therapist. Did either sex and/or gender influence your career decision?

Chapters 11, 12 and 13 will discuss sociological theories in relation to organizations, professions and work in more detail. It is useful to raise the question here, in a chapter concerning sex and gender, of why so many women, but so few men, enter the profession of occupational therapy. Issues concerning sex and gender have a place within the wider debate of work, in the notion of 'women's work' and 'men's work', for example. We are also reminded that the 'separation of workplace and household led to the ideology embodied in the statement that a woman's place is in the home' (Primeau 1992).

Others, for example Litterst (1992), have highlighted issues such as the origin and development of occupational therapy and how this was influenced by ideas about appropriate work for women. She draws attention to an ideology dominant in the late nineteenth and early twentieth centuries that saw women as being nurturing and caring. Some women were able to turn this ideology to their advantage as the need for 're-construction aides' (p. 20) resulting from World War I gave them the opportunity to acquire high-status work outside the home, albeit still within the context of nurturing and caring. It must be remembered that this was only the case for middle-class women. Indeed, one Boston newspaper of the time described the new occupational therapy students as 'society girls'. Thus although, in one sense, some women subjectively experienced these new opportunities as liberating, they were objectively still subject to male power and ideology.

FEMINIST CRITIQUES OF SOCIOLOGY

A criticism of sociology, until comparatively recently, was that it was dominated by male values and unrepresentative of social reality. Abbott & Wallace (1990, p. 1), writing from a particular feminist perspective, argue that sociology is a male-dominated discipline. They further argue

that 'while malestream sociological theory can no longer ignore feminist perspectives it has tended to marginalise them.' This critique stimulated a movement within radical sociology to incorporate feminist perspectives and examine the position of women in society. It has had a bearing not only on the analysis of social inequality, but also upon the nature and type of research carried out within social science. Richardson & Robinson (1993, p. 5) remind us of the role of feminist theory within women's studies, in that it seeks to address the fact that individual disciplines, in the context here sociology, are 'gender blind – presenting male values and experience as human ones'. The concept of phallocentrism is important to this critique of sociology and refers to the way in which woman is always defined *in relation to* man. This concept is also reflected in the English language, in which we can see in the words female and woman the way in which women are seen to be an adjunct to men.

Feminist theory

The word 'feminism' has been used throughout this section, and it is important now to consider the term and its meanings. The 'taxonomy' of Marxist or socialist, liberal and radical, previously used concerning feminism, and outlined in Chapter 2, is thought by some to be too limiting in the late 1990s. Feminist theory can be seen as developing as a reaction to and a critique of theoretical 'malestreams' such as sociology, but its influence is also to be seen in history, politics, literature, psychology, philosophy and many other subject areas and disciplines. It is, of course, not possible here fully to develop and theoretically debate the various strands of feminism not the subsequent academic development of women's studies. We are, however, reminded of the importance of feminism by Humm (1992), who states that 'in this century, it is feminism which represents *the* major change in social thinking and politics because only feminism *radically* questions an understanding of "men" and "women" and the social structures which maintain their differences' (original emphasis). This statement emphasizes the socialization process of learned gender role, referred to earlier. Humm also reminds us that what has been called second-wave feminism addresses psychoanalysis, poststructuralism and postmodernism. A major feature of feminism is that it reminds us that there is space for the development of new theories and new knowledge.

Developments in feminist theory

It is important at this point to note the existence of 'feminist perspectives'; i.e. a plurality of feminisms exists. Tong's (1992, p. 7) thoughts emphasize this plurality; she notes:

That feminism is many and not one is to be expected because women are many and not one. The more feminist thoughts we have, the better. By refusing to centre, congeal, and cement their separate thoughts into a unified truth too inflexible to change, feminists resist patriarchal dogma.

This statement by Tong reflects a more recent development within feminism, which may be described as anti-essentialist.

Anti-essentialism

We noted earlier how biological essentialism appealed to universalism or the idea of a basic human nature. The term 'essentialism' has also been used to describe a view that sees all women as having the same interests and experiences. This view was typical of some feminists in the 1960s and 70s. More recent feminist writers, such as Spelman (1990), have argued that feminist analysis cannot isolate sex and gender from issues such as class and race. Feminists writing within this perspective would want to debate such questions as whether a black South African woman under apartheid had more in common with a black South African man than with a white woman. Similarly, as highlighted in Chapter 15, disabled women have been critical of the way in which non-disabled women have looked at community care. Thus anti-essentialism argues that while all women may share some interests and experiences, there are also important differences between women belonging to different social groups and cultures.

The discussion so far has considered sex, gender, femininity and masculinity. Debates regarding biological determinism and social construction, including the nature/nurture debate, remain central to most feminist perspectives. With this in mind, you should now be able to articulate the complexity surrounding the difference between sex and gender. We have also considered the notion of a 'caring profession' and the possibility that we ascribe notions of sex and/or gender to this term. That is to say, 'caring profession' can be construed as a gendered term.

At this point, it important to consider the implications for occupational therapy of what has been discussed so far.

ISSUES FOR OCCUPATIONAL THERAPY

Contemporary feminism, despite its growth, remains at the margins. The issue of why occupational therapists, who, as we have noted, are predominantly women, have not embraced feminist perspectives into theory and practice is interesting. This question has been raised by writers in occupational therapy, such as Hamlin et al (1992), Miller (1992) and Frank (1992).

This part of the chapter will now explore implications for the practice of occupational therapy involving debates within this complex area. Although many of the issues have resonance within the totality of the caring professions, literature from occupational therapy will mainly be examined in an attempt to explore aspects that have been considered salient to a profession concerned with occupational behaviour and its dynamics.

The following aspects will be covered:

- historical influences on occupational therapy
- occupational therapy as a 'female, caring profession'
- sex role-stereotyping within the practice of occupational therapy
- current debates around the feminine principle in occupational therapy.

HISTORICAL INFLUENCES

On both sides of the Atlantic, occupational therapy emerged at a time when women were striving for greater equality with men, and, as Kelly (1996) notes, the history of the profession is closely interwoven with the development of feminist ideas. The evolution of occupational therapy is replete with indomitable women, usually from middle- and upper middle-class backgrounds, who sought to demonstrate the ways in which involvement in meaningful and purposeful activity contributed towards rehabilitation and health.

> **Activity 6.7**
>
> Spend some time tracing the origins of occupational therapy within your own context. Who were the prime movers in establishing centres where people could learn to be occupational therapists?

In an American context, Litterst (1992) explores the role of value systems and ideology, which stimulated the emergence of occupational therapy. She notes that 'industrial organisation and family values combined as influences on the initial form of the work of occupational therapy in the context of war'. This is a valuable comment on American society, which she believes was, at the time, experiencing an antimodernist movement that reacted against the implications of industrial organization. The antimodernist movement fuelled a wish for social reform, and Adolf Meyer (1922) paralleled this view in his belief and thrust towards the natural basis and balance of activities in work, play, rest and sleep. Thus the shape and nature of the profession of occupational therapy evolved. Taking a slightly different route, Frank (1992) traces the history of occupational therapy in feminist terms and reveals the sources of gender segregation in occupational therapy. She considers that sex role-stereotyping has had a powerful impact on the emergence and maintenance of occupational therapy as a women's profession. Nevertheless, bearing in mind the anti-essentialist debate, it is worth noting the exclusion and stratification within the profession on the basis of race, class and dis-

ability. This has given rise to current drives within the profession in the mid 1990s to recruit from wider ethnic, socioeconomic and other groups.

> **Activity 6.8**
>
> Consider your context. What is the ratio of men to women in your year? Discuss reasons for the disproportionate number of females to males.

OCCUPATIONAL THERAPY AS A GENDERED PROFESSION

In a British context, Cracknell (1989) examined factors within the health service that continued to polarize the position of men and women, such as the dominance of the medical profession and the nature of professionalization. This work was an important forerunner to examinations of what constitutes the 'feminine principle' within research, clinical reasoning, education and the current practice of occupational therapy. Like others within female-dominated professions, Cracknell believes that the feminist perspective could contribute to a deeper analysis and understanding of both therapeutic intervention and research.

Cracknell (1989, p. 386) reminds us that occupational therapy 'emerged at a time when women were struggling for greater equality with men, following the gradual reduction of their freedom of the previous 200 years'. Many other factors will, of course, influence any debate regarding 'equality', and the issue of essentialism, as discussed earlier, must be borne in mind. Age, class, ethnic origin, education, childhood and sexuality will be some of the issues that might have an influence. Cracknell further reminds us of the stereotypical 'characteristics' of girls and boys, some of which were alluded to earlier in this chapter. However, she acknowledges a situation in which women have been defined as 'other' within a male hegemony (the domination of male ideas and interests). Thus, in modern industrial societies, we see the devaluing of the 'feminine' and the promotion of the 'rational', 'scientific' and competitive. Feminist perspectives on medicine, occupation and the professions are offered by Cracknell as being a helpful way forward in order to understand the limitations within women's professions and careers.

Individuals may, of course, feel that a sex equality debate is inappropriate within a profession such as occupational therapy; but it might be useful to consider the aforementioned discussion and consider a phrase such as 'career man'?

Activity 6.9

What are your first thoughts on reading the phrase 'career man'? It may be useful to consider why the term 'career woman' is more commonly used before attempting to answer the question posed here.

Feminist theorists would argue that assigned and learned gender roles are limiting for women in relation to work and occupational choices. At this point it is useful to reflect on the previous discussion related to sex, gender and feminism. The question of occupational therapy as one of the 'caring' professions will be considered.

Perceptions of caring within the profession

The analysis of caring by social science highlights how heavy the term is with value-laden perceptions. Caring professions have traditionally been stereotypically considered as an extension of women's work and were, as such, afforded lower status. Feminine qualities appeared synonymous with those of therapy in terms of someone who valued the client, listened and was nonjudgmental. Devereaux (1984, p. 798), in discussing the elements of the therapeutic relationship, informs us that occupational therapists are concerned about caring and that as a group, they have 'superb skills for developing and tending caring relationships'. One wonders whether she is unconsciously drawing on notions of occupational therapy as female profession. Sachs & Labovitz (1994) remind us of the gendered nature of the care versus cure debate. Thus caring tasks are assigned predominantly to and assumed by women, a low value being placed on such caring, against a higher value attributed to curing, which is associated with the traditionally male-dominated medical profession. Here again, we see the devaluing of what might be considered to be within the feminine domain.

If caring is defined as women's work, what meaning does this have for a profession comprising both women and men? Taylor (1995) reminds us that occupational therapy, in addition to nursing and social work, is one of those professions which developed from the tasks and skills that were (and to some extent still are) construed in the West as the responsibility of women. Taylor's (1995) analysis draws attention to the difference inherent in caring 'about' a client and caring 'for', which requires a level of intimacy consistent with Gilligan's ethic of care that is attributable to women. Taylor's work is, however, offered here as an interesting introduction to complicated debates regarding Gilligan's work, sociological debates, feminist debates and concepts of work, the professions and caring.

Gilligan's ethic of care

The work of Gilligan (1982) is useful in that it explores the differences between how women and men define themselves and approach moral reasoning within a context of caring. This work explored different kinds of moral development and contrasted them to the influential work of Kohlberg (1969), which, in her view, focused exclusively on how men thought and behaved.

Gilligan revealed how immersed women were in attempting to fulfil the needs of others and the importance to them of relationships. Many writers have commented upon and critiqued Gilligan's work (Dunlop 1986, Puka 1990, Tronto 1987). While offering interesting and challenging insights regarding the theories and social construction of care, she incurred criticism for basing her work on white, middle-class women. It must also be stated that Gilligan's position is contradictory in feminist terms as her research raises debates related to biological essentialism and the nature/nurture debate, in her ascribing of roles and in stating that it is 'natural' for women to care.

In addition to Taylor, other writers, for example Primeau (1992), Frank (1992), Mathewson (1975) and Miller (1992), have offered feminist critiques of the notions of work, gender segregation and occupational therapy as a profession.

SEX ROLE-STEREOTYPING WITHIN THE PRACTICE OF OCCUPATIONAL THERAPY

As noted in Chapter 5, a role is, to a greater or lesser extent (depending on whether you take a functionalist or an interactionist perspective), largely determined by other people's expectations. Every society makes certain distinctions about the roles that are attributed to men and women. This appears more evident in some cultures, for example Islam, than in others. In Western cultures, on the other hand, much of our behaviour is assumed to be increasingly free of sex role expectations, although some feminists would question this. Nevertheless, stereotypes do exist and can influence education, employment and opportunities within health care.

One of the most notable writers concerned with this aspect within occupational therapy is Bracegirdle (1991a,b,c), who, in writing in a British context, explores the socially constructed stereotypes of women, particularly within mental health. In a trilogy of articles, she examined how prevalent male predominance was within the psychiatric profession and that sex role-stereotyping in particular had a distinct influence on the diagnosis of depression.

In examining the emphasis on sex-differentiated activities for women, she outlines the seeming collusion of occupational therapy in maintaining stereotypes. Reviewing literature in the *British Journal of Occupational Therapy* over a period of 24 years, however, she detected a slight shift to less traditional roles and tasks that were offered as therapeutic activity. Nevertheless, in a small study into the prescription of activities for men and women, she found an adherence to traditional sex role-differentiated activities. In the interesting discussion that accompanied this work, students voiced concerns about offering non-traditional activities at times when clients were feeling vulnerable. Nevertheless, Bracegirdle urges therapists not to undermine a healthy wish to reject traditional roles and to have on offer a range of possibilities to allow all people equal access to valued activities. The key message is that occupational therapists need to be mindful of the way in which they construe activities and to reflect upon the possibility of reinforcing gender-related stereotypes.

Activity 6.10

To what extent was gender a factor in the choice of activities offered to men and women in your last fieldwork placement?

In a very different context, Jessop (1993) outlines the contribution of occupational therapy in facilitating the transition of a male-to-female transsexual within the domain of life skills. The chosen gender role requires the therapist to explore with the client the perception and expectations of the female role. While possibilities do exist for reinforcing traditional sex role-stereotypes, the nature of client-centred therapy is such that people who are in this position are encouraged to explore and choose their own interpretation of gender. Work of this type also challenges the therapist to explore the whole notion of sexuality.

We saw earlier in this chapter how gender is socially constructed; in the same way, we can question the supposed 'naturalness' of heterosexual relationships. For occupational therapists, this means being aware of their own and other people's responses to gay, lesbian or bisexual clients. It means being prepared to consider that a social skills programme for people with learning disabilities should also incorporate the possibility of gay/lesbian as well as heterosexual relationships. Also open to question are notions of dominance and submissiveness within sexual relationships and the double standards that are attached to men's sexual behaviour compared with that of women. Thus a man who has many sexual partners is considered to be 'a bit of a lad', whereas a woman may be 'cheap' or 'easy'.

THE FEMININE PRINCIPLE AND OCCUPATIONAL THERAPY

The notion of a synchrony or balance between

masculine and feminine poles is prevalent in psychology, philosophy and anthropology. Nevertheless, men have maintained the dominant position in society for thousands of years, either by physical force or through the power of ideology. This has influenced all aspects of life, particularly science and research, in which 'hard science' is associated with quantitative methods and is deemed superior to 'soft science', which is found in more qualitative approaches and is still viewed with scepticism in some scientific disciplines.

What has become known as the 'feminine principle' is an acknowledgement of the values, actions and worth of attributes such as intuition, nurturance and compassion, as noted by Kelly (1996). Occupational therapy is still ambivalent about wholeheartedly embracing this as a value system and frequently attempts to emulate scientific respectability by attempting to measure its practice in a strictly controlled manner. A recurring issue within the occupational therapy literature is a concern with the development of standardized assessments. If the features that draw people to the profession are associated with engaging people in a process that moves towards growth and personal change and are not measurable or directly open to standardized outcome measures, the profession is in a conceptual conundrum. It is torn between one set of values and another.

Kelly (1996) suggests that a 'gender identity crisis' exists, whereby, on the one hand, the pro-

fession favours holism as a basic value but on the other, aligns itself with the powerful biomedical model or masculine principle for referred power and influence. In Kelly's analysis, attention is drawn to patriarchal attitudes that pervade the educational curriculum of occupational therapy, for example where reference lists seldom include a feminist text.

CONCLUSION

This chapter has sought to explain, explore and define issues of sex, gender and feminism within occupational therapy practice. These three areas may not at first seem relevant within sociological debates and current theories and practice within the profession of occupational therapy. However, the importance of applying feminist perspectives to these issues in order fully to understand the limits and constraints that may be placed upon some professions, within a hegemony such as medicine, has been stressed. Professions that are composed largely of women are controlled and constrained within such a system.

The importance of understanding social construction related to the terms 'femininity' and 'masculinity' has been raised, and issues related to role and sex role-stereotyping have been addressed. Caring and notions of 'women's work' and 'men's work' have been recognized as issues for continuing and further debate within sociology and occupational therapy. Feminist perspectives have been offered as one way forward in understanding why some professions, commonly those in which women work, are defined as 'caring' professions. The implications of this for both women and men have been highlighted.

Activity 6.11

Consider what attracted you to the profession of occupational therapy. What qualities or values did you feel were part of the job?

REFERENCES

Abbott P, Wallace C 1990 An introduction to sociology. Feminist perspectives. Routledge, London

Bracegirdle H 1991a The female stereotype and occupational therapy for women with depression. British Journal of Occupational Therapy 54(5): 193–194

Bracegirdle H 1991b Two hundred years of therapeutic occupations for women hospital patients. British Journal of Occupational Therapy 54(6): 231–232

Bracegirdle H 1991c Occupational therapy. Students' choice of gender differentiated activities for psychiatric patients. British Journal of Occupational Therapy 54(7): 266–268

Cracknell E 1989 Conflicts for the female therapist: some

reflections. British Journal of Occupational Therapy 52(10): 386–388

de Beauvoir S 1976 The second sex. Penguin, Harmondsworth

Devereaux E B 1984 Occupational therapy's challenge: the caring relationship. American Journal of Occupational Therapy 38(12): 791–798

Dunlop M J 1986 Is a science of caring possible? Journal of Advanced Nursing 11: 661–670

Eitzen D S 1980 Social Problems Allyn and Bacon, Boston

Frank G 1992 Opening feminist histories of occupational therapy. American Journal of Occupational Therapy 46(11): 989–999

Gilligan C 1982 In a different voice. Harvard University Press, NY

Hamlin R B, Loukas K M, Froehlich J, MacRae N 1992 Feminism: an inclusion perspective. American Journal of Occupational Therapy 46(1): 967–970

Humm M (ed.) 1992 Feminisms. A reader. Harvester Wheatsheaf, Hertfordshire

Jessop N 1993 Occupational therapy with a male to female transexual. A case study. British Journal of Occupational Therapy 56(9): 989–999

Kelly G 1996 Feminist or feminine? The feminine principle in occupational therapy. British Journal of Occupational Therapy 59(1): 2–6

Kohlberg L 1969 Stage and sequence. The cognitive developmental approach to socialisation. In: Goslin D A (ed) Handbook of socialisation theory and research. Rand McNally, Chicago

Levin W C 1988 Sociological ideas concepts and applications. Wadsworth Publications, Belmont, CA

Litterst T A 1992 Occupational therapy: the role of ideology in the development of a profession for women. American Journal of Occupational Therapy 46(1): 20–25

Madoc-Jones B, Coates J (eds) 1996 An introduction to women's studies. Blackwell, Oxford

Mathewson M 1975 Female and married. Damaging to the profession? American Journal of Occupational Therapy 29(10): 601–605

Meyer A 1922 The philosophy of occupational therapy. Archives of occupational therapy 1(1): 1–10

Miller R J 1992 Interwoven threads: occupational therapy, feminism, and holistic health. American Journal of Occupational Therapy 46(11): 1013–1019

Oakley A 1985 Sex, gender and society. Gower / Maurice TempleSmith, Hampshire

Primeau L A 1992 Woman's place: unpaid work in the home. American Journal of Occupational Therapy 46(11): 981–988

Puka B 1990 The liberation of caring; a different voice for Gilligan's 'different voice'. Hypatia 5(1): 58–82

Richardson D, Robinson V (eds) 1993 Introducing women's studies. Macmillan, London

Sachs D, Labovitz D R 1994 The caring occupational therapist: scope of professional role boundaries. American Journal of Occupational Therapy 48(11): 997–1005

Spelman E 1990 Inessential woman. Women's Press, London

Stacey J 1983 Sexuality and male dominance. In: Richardson D, Robinson V (eds) Introducing women's studies. Macmillan, London

Taylor J 1995 A different voice in occupational therapy. British Journal of Occupational Therapy 58(4): 170–174

Tong R 1992 Feminist thought. A comprehensive introduction. Routledge, London

Tronto J C 1987 Beyond gender difference to a theory of care. Signs 12(4): 644–663

7

Multicultural society

Isabel Dyck

LIVING IN A MULTICULTURAL SOCIETY

Contemporary advanced industrial societies are characterized by culturally diverse populations. Although the movement of people around the world is not new, the development of a global economy, enormous advances in communications technology and political unrest have resulted in extensive international flows of people and goods in recent decades. As people are dislocated and resettle, whether through processes of immigration, refugee resettlement, migrant labour or business investment, the cultural and physical landscapes of cities and towns change. In larger cities, for example, it is commonplace to see newspapers from around the world, restaurants offering the foods of India, Mexico, Vietnam and other distant places, branches of overseas banks, and foods from diverse cultures on grocery store shelves. Depending on the city, there may be speciality stores selling saris, or corner stores run by immigrants from Iraq or Hong Kong. Where there is a long history of settlement from China, an established 'Chinatown' area often exists. Countries with native or aboriginal populations, such as Australia, Canada, New Zealand and the USA, have an added layer of diversity to their society.

Economic conditions, immigration policies and colonial and political ties all contribute to patterns of movement and resettlement, and affect the jobs that people do, the places immigrants come to live in and the positioning of native peoples in society. The cultural diversity of contemporary societies therefore reflects the outcome of a complexity of social, economic and political linkages and processes that have been generated over time. While such societies have distinctive features relating to their unique social and political histories, there are also common patterns that have attracted the interest of sociologists and other social scientists. One is the persistence of the cultural distinctiveness of some immigrant groups over several generations, the other a tendency for such groups to occupy different class positions in a 'vertical mosaic', a term coined by Porter (1965) in the Canadian context. At the top of the hierarchy are commonly people of white Anglo-Saxon origin, with 'black' or native peoples at the bottom. A group's position in the vertical mosaic is accompanied by different access to resources, such as education, health care, housing or employment opportunities and political representation.

Activity 7.1

Think about the place where you live or grew up. What signs of cultural diversity are evident to you? Do you know the history of immigrant settlement of that community? How have immigration policies influenced its current cultural composition?

SOCIOLOGICAL THEORIES OF CULTURAL DIVERSITY: THE DYNAMICS OF ETHNICITY AND 'RACE'

The continued inequality of ethnic or racial groups in multicultural society, in addition to class and gender differentials, has been a particular concern for sociological investigation. Sociology has examined such questions as:

- How do we explain the continuing differential access to resources, power and prestige on ethnic and racial lines?
- How can we best understand ethnic distinctiveness and the relationships between culturally diverse groups?
- How is the 'difference' of culture organized in

everyday life; what is culture and what is its relationship to ethnicity and race?

Culture

Culture is a complex phenomenon that defies easy definition. Common among concepts of culture, however, is the idea of shared meanings through which members of a culture interact and communicate with each other. Shared meanings involve ideas, concepts and knowledge, and include the beliefs, values and norms that shape standards and rules of behaviour as people go about their everyday lives. Culture also refers to the material forms that reflect ideas and modes of thinking, such as everyday and ceremonial objects, the built environment, foods, dress and the visual and performing arts. Such ideas, knowledge and customary ways of behaving are transmitted from generation to generation through socialization.

The notion that culture, as a set of ideas, concepts and knowledge, acts as a framework for interpreting experience and guiding behaviour is widely accepted. The relationship between culture and behaviour, however, is not clear cut. A traditional functionalist view tends to emphasize the stability of culture, its learnt nature and its internalization, which act to the advantage of its participants and order in society. People are viewed as carriers or repositories of culture, and cultural 'blueprints' for action are understood to be highly predictive of behaviour. In its extreme form, this association between cultural ideals and behaviour is known as cultural determinism. That is, if we know about a person's culture, we can anticipate what sort of actions he or she is likely to take in a given situation.

Subcultures

Variations in the standards and behaviours of a culture based on, for example, age, local geography and occupational groupings may exist and are termed subcultures. Members of subcultures share a subset of values and meanings, which may be signalled by outward forms such as distinctive dress, food habits and specific jargon that set the group apart. Youth gangs, students, professions and ethnic groups may all be considered subgroups in society with distinctive behaviours or norms but who also share some of the dominant values of society. While this approach acknowledges that cultural blueprints can change over time, for example as an immigrant adjusts to a new society, and that there may be subcultural variation, human beings are understood as cultural products rather than makers of culture.

Cultural variation

A rigid culturalist perspective is challenged by a conceptualization of culture that emphasizes its mutability, or openness to change. An accumulation of anthropological research shows that ideas and knowledge, and their associated meanings, are not fixed but constantly undergo negotiation during the course of everyday social interaction (see for example Geertz 1983, Hannerz 1992, Keesing 1987). The 'cultural repertoire' of an individual can incorporate new possibilities for action as new events are experienced and social change occurs. Rather than focusing on the socialization of people into a culture, with an emphasis on its ongoing transmission and stability, this approach sees culture as fluid and constantly being remade. Subcultural variation is interpreted differently, shifting attention away from a focus on the group expression of different values, to the differential access to power and knowledge in society of its different members. The transmission of cultural ideas and knowledge is not even, so that not all meanings are known to all members of society. For example, members of certain professions have access to specialized knowledge and language that are not available to the lay person. Furthermore, meanings that are dominant in society may be understood and drawn upon in different ways in guiding action and making sense of everyday life. One's age, gender or class position could be influential factors. Culture therefore presents a range of possible ways of acting in the world rather than determining behaviour.

Ethnicity and race

Just as the concept of culture has developed, so too the concepts of ethnicity and race have been used in different ways in the three main sociological approaches that have been used in the analyses of culturally diverse societies. These are:

- a traditional functionalist approach
- a structural approach informed by Marxism
- a social constructionist perspective.

Each approach employs a different way of understanding the relationship between culture, ethnicity and race that influences its interpretation of the dynamics of cultural diversity in society.

TRADITIONAL FUNCTIONALIST APPROACHES

Theories of cultural change and ethnic persistence in functionalist approaches tend to emphasize order and harmony in society. Ethnicity is a core concept in explanation and is closely related to a notion of culture that emphasizes its internalization through socialization. It refers to a sense of belonging and loyalty to a group of common national and cultural heritage. Members of an ethnic group share descent, language, traditions, religion and other common cultural features and experiences that distinguish them from other groups. While ethnicity refers primarily to self-identification with an ethnic group, ethnic identification is also used by others in society in making intergroup distinctions. In functionalist theory, explanations of ethnic group persistence in society rely heavily on the idea of a person's primary identification with a cultural community or ethnic group. A core common culture is important to societal order in functionalist theory. Models of society have focused on how ethnic loyalties may change over time or may be managed to reduce conflict, for example through assimilation.

Assimilation model

The notion of the assimilation of immigrant ethnic groups into the majority culture had an influential advocate in Robert Park of the Chicago School of Sociology in the USA. It is based on the idea that immigrants become more like the majority culture over time as they lose their ethnic distinctiveness and subscribe to majority cultural ideas and practices. In the case of the USA the majority culture to which immigrant groups are expected to assimilate is predominantly Anglo-Saxon in character. This model suggests that groups first become culturally assimilated, or acculturated, as they learn to speak English and adopt 'mainstream' ways, and then become structurally assimilated. That is, individuals become fully integrated into society, participating in all aspects of its social, economic and political life, ethnicity losing its importance in self- or group identification.

Amalgamation model: the 'melting pot'

The idea of the melting pot is popularly thought of as characteristic of North American society and is a version of the assimilation argument. In this model, rather than ethnic groups integrating through assimilation to the dominant culture, all groups are part of a process that synthesizes a variety of cultures. As the term melting pot suggests, the theory is that all ethnic groups contribute to the institutions and identity of a young nation. The resulting amalgam resembles something different from its constituent parts. Specific ethnic groups do not remain distinct, but valued features from different cultures are adopted in creating a unique and new culture.

Pluralism and the ethnic mosaic

A further model that falls within a broadly functionalist understanding of society is that of an ethnic mosaic, reflecting the cultural pluralism of a country's population. Distinct cultural groups live side by side, interacting together as part of a single society and subscribing to its central values and goals. In this model, there is, therefore, an assumption of some sharing of common culture, relative equality among groups and a mutual tolerance of the differences between them, such as each other's religion, language and family organization. Common participation in the economic and political life of the nation is accompanied by a maintenance of cultural distinctiveness in the private aspects of everyday life. The cultural distinctiveness will, however, be in a modified form compared with the traditional cultural identities (Glazer & Moynihan 1963).

> **Activity 7.2**
>
> From your own knowledge and observations, how well do you think any of the above models match the society in which you live? What sort of evidence might suggest a less than ideal fit?

Barriers to integration

Both the assimilation and amalgamation theories of cultural change are based on an evolutionary model of society. The idea is that urbanization and technological change, as the source of universal values of rationality and science, promote cultural homogeneity. Both models view cultural conformity as the key to reducing conflict between ethnic groups and maintaining order in society. The idea of an ethnic mosaic also stresses harmony and order, and has been promoted in Canada through a multicultural policy recognizing the cultural pluralism of the population and the right of people to express their ethnic identity and develop institutions to maintain it. In reality, however, these ideals of society are not met. There is continued evidence of conflict between ethnic groups and a persistence of ethnic and racial inequalities. Ethnocentrism of majority culture members, and stereotyping and prejudice against ethnic groups, act as barriers to integration and cause ongoing tensions between groups.

The traditional functionalist approach is criticized for its overemphasis on culture as a determinant of action and its neglect of the structural positions of different groups that constrain their participation in society. For example, the entrenchment of black–white relations in the USA and of British race relations cannot be adequately explained without consideration of their historical context and the legacy of colonial relations. Functionalist models also cannot adequately incorporate the experience of aboriginal or native peoples who have consistently occupied the lowest position in stratified societies. Their story is one of their legal, political and economic oppression. Loss of traditional lands and different citizenship rights occurred as native peoples came under the jurisdiction of the colonial government, whether in Australia, Canada, New Zealand or the USA, to the detriment of their economies and social organization. Their exclusion from full participation in the institutions of the majority culture has resulted in their subordination and marginalization in society.

Traditional functionalist approaches seem to lack any analysis of power relations. An alternative approach would be to view differential access to housing, jobs and education in terms of a group's location in social structures.

STRUCTURAL MARXIST APPROACH

A class analysis informed by Marxism presents an alternative approach to understanding cultural diversity in contemporary Western societies. Exploring the relationship between class, ethnicity and race is of key importance. Unlike traditional functionalism, a structural Marxist perspective sees race and ethnic divisions as functional to capitalism. Racism, which entertains the idea of the biological superiority of a white race, maintains such divisions and is itself a product of capitalist expansion through colonialism. For example, in the British context, the phenomenon of the continued marginalization of immigrants from former colonies, particularly those with darker skin colour from the Caribbean and the Indian subcontinent, is explained in terms of the class relations of capitalist society.

In Marxist theory, the different relationship to the mode of production of the owners of capital and the workers, whose labour is purchased by the owners, is understood to be the basis of social class. Inequalities of income and power derive from the different relationships of groups to the mode of production and control over capital.

These result in different class interests and conflict. Although ethnic and racial minorities are part of the working class, they are distinguished on the basis of race from the white members of the working class, forming what is termed a class fraction. As a result of racism, the working class remains disunited, thus reducing the threat of their collective action against their capitalist oppressors. Hence social control is maintained. Furthermore, ethnic and racial groups are relegated to marginal positions in society, providing a supply of labour for menial jobs, to the advantage of the workings of capitalism. While this theory of 'divide and rule' simplifies the complex nature of class relations and their intersection with ethnicity, a class-informed analysis of ethnic and race relations continues to hold considerable appeal as a basis for political action.

A modified form of the above argument recognizes the complexity of relationships between immigrant minorities and the white majority. Rex's (1970, 1986) influential work on race relations also recognizes class as important in understanding divisions among ethnic and racial minorities but emphasizes competition over scarce resources in a class society. He also points out that although race, ethnicity and social class tend to overlap, their boundaries do not necessarily exactly coincide. Discrimination on racial grounds results in job segregation, wage differentials, differential access to housing and health care, and other unequal treatment. Such discrimination is key to understanding the structural position of minority groups in society. Rex notes that all ethnic minorities are not disadvantaged to the same extent and may hold different occupational positions in the mode of production. Ethnicity, however, is always a disadvantage for one of the groups.

The focus on race relations suggests that ethnic

Activity 7.3

Think about the minority groups in your society. Which groups were the subjects of colonial expansion? Are there specific groups that appear to be disadvantaged in terms of employment, housing, education and health?

persistence and tensions between groups cannot be reduced to cultural preferences and ethnic group loyalty but need to be understood within a framework of the class relations of society. Yet there are difficulties with structural Marxist theory as it tends to cast members of minority groups as pawns in economic processes, neglecting the capacity of groups to organize politically. Although later formulations recognize that ethnic and racial minorities do not form a homogeneous class fraction, class struggle predominates as the key factor. Class relations and racial discrimination are important in understanding the differential access of ethnic minorities to power and material resources in society. However, further thinking about the concepts of ethnicity and race stresses their socially constructed nature, not only within relations of class, but also in the context of everyday social practices.

SOCIAL CONSTRUCTIONIST APPROACHES

Social constructionism is an approach developed from the early work of Berger & Luckmann (1967), who were concerned with how knowledge and reality are constructed in the course of everyday social interaction. This approach emphasizes that there are no 'natural' ethnic or racial characteristics but only attributions of certain characteristics to particular groups that are explained in terms of ethnicity or race. Scientists have found that there are more genetic similarities between 'blacks' and 'whites' than within these categories. Despite this, people continue to think of certain groups as having particular, biologically determined, characteristics, such as dishonesty or violence, or temperaments suiting them to particular types of work. In Britain, for example, stereotypical notions of the manual dexterity and docility of Asian women have played a part in particular hiring practices in the textile industry. In rejecting this type of thinking, known as essentialism, some authors use single quotation marks around the word 'race' to signal that the concept does not indicate a real entity but is instead an idea that only exists within the context of social relationships.

Social constructionists are interested in how everyday, social practices construct meanings about perceived differences between people and frame the experiences of groups categorized in terms of ethnicity or race. Many informal and administrative practices affect what men and women immigrants do and where they live. What may at first sight seem to be the exercise of cultural preference or the 'natural' abilities of a group can be better understood as the social construction of an ethnic or racial minority. The dynamics of social interaction at the micro level is therefore the central focus.

In Canada, for example, many women from 'non-traditional' source countries, such as India or Hong Kong, have entered Canada in the immigrant categories of 'family class' or assisted relative', which do not give them government-sponsored access to job training programmes, language training and supported childcare. This makes it difficult for them to upgrade previous job-related skills or acquire new ones more appropriate for the Canadian labour market. Many work as berry-pickers, in restaurant kitchens, as hospital cleaners or in the garment industry, often finding work through word-of-mouth contacts. Their association with particular sectors of the economy tends to solidify over time. As a result, perceptions of what work certain groups suit and do well at feeds back into hiring practices.

CONCEPTUAL CONUNDRUMS

Although the socially constructed character of ethnicity and race has been recognized in sociology for several decades, a tendency to reify ethnic and racial categories remains. In Britain, 'Black' and 'Asian' are common designators of broad groupings of people, while in the USA, the categories of Hispanic, Black and Native American are commonly used in comparative studies and in the collection of census data. The 'hyphenated' Canadian has entered the politics of language, with more recent immigrant groups such as the 'Indo-Canadians' joining the founding English- and French-Canadian groups. This produces a conundrum, for if such categorizations have no theoretical validity as descriptions of 'natural' differences between groups but continue to be used in explaining the social world, are they then contributing to the idea that they are actually real?

Racism and racialization

Miles (1993) suggests that the continued use of the concept of race by sociologists, such as in 'race relations studies', inadvertently reaffirms the notion of the existence of race despite the recognition of its social construction. Instead, he focuses on racism and racialization, emphasizing the power of the idea of race and discourses about it in affecting people's life chances and their position in society. Racism is commonly used to refer to both a discourse about race that legitimizes inequality between groups of people viewed as biologically or culturally distinct, and everyday social interactions that result in the differential treatment of such groups. The specific content of ideas about race, however, is not necessarily confined to a context of social relations defined in terms of 'blackness' and 'whiteness'. For example, the Irish used to be thought of as a separate race in Britain, and there may be racism among non-white groups. Important to the notion of racism, however, is that certain physical features or an idea of 'natural' cultural characteristics are negatively evaluated.

Although racism is often thought of as an individual attitude or belief, which may or may not lead to specific discriminatory action, the concept of institutional racism is also important in constructing inequalities. Organizational practices may be built into the everyday operation of major institutions, tending to exclude subordinate groups or act to their disadvantage.

Closely linked to the concept of racism is that of racialization. This refers to the process or, more accurately, a complexity of social, economic, political and ideological processes by which people come to be designated as a certain category, such as 'black', which then has ongoing consequences for their life experiences. A racialized group is one that been constructed as different from other groups through the effects

of a discourse that draws on biological and cultural 'markers' in describing and rationalizing the group's different social, economic and political position in society. The concept of racialization is useful in that it avoids the use of the concept of race, which suggests its real existence, while still acknowledging that ideas about race are drawn on as people make social differentiations in understanding the world around them, and affect the life opportunities of different groups.

Activity 7.4

How convincing is the argument of racialization, compared with that of a structural Marxist approach, in explaining the subordination of minority groups?

Awareness of the power of representations of what people are like or how they experience their lives has led to further thinking about the links between culture, identity and the organization of difference in society. The ways in which certain groups are represented in the media, in art, in novels, in popular and academic writing and in ways of talking about race can all contribute to the 'naturalizing' of difference through a rationale of ethnicity and race. Not all images and discourses portray minority groups in negative ways, but we are all aware of news reports of Asian gangs, accounts of 'black' crime rates or other 'facts' that construct images of certain groups that both discount the diversity within groups and tell us little of the contexts of the 'facts'. Whatever the reason for race, rather than age, gender or class position, being chosen as a main descriptor, such representations become part and parcel of processes of racialization. They enter the stock of ideas and knowledge through which we make sense of the world.

Activity 7.5

Think about the images you hold of certain minority groups. What sources of knowledge do you draw on in constructing these images? Think of a particular minority group and its representation in different media.

Differences in disadvantage

Much sociological analysis focuses on the discourses and practices of the majority culture and tends to emphasize exclusionary practices and processes of subordination on both an individual and an institutional level. Yet racialized groups are heterogeneous, and not all members are disadvantaged in the same way. The wealthy 'investor class' immigrant from Hong Kong living in Canada, for example, enjoys a very different position in society from that of the widow from China who entered in the 'family class' category, yet both may be categorized as 'Orientals'. In Britain, there are differences in levels of unemployment between Asians and Afro-Caribbeans. Similarly, the diversity within 'whiteness' is rarely addressed in discussions of racialization. This is not to dismiss the powerful effects of racism but to be wary of explaining all experiences in terms of it. Miles (1989), for example, states that while unemployment rates are higher for people of Caribbean origin in Britain, they tend to be employed in sectors of the economy that are vulnerable to downturns in the economy. People are positioned in society in different ways, within local geographies and economies, and within a complexity of relationships, including those of gender and age. In practice, it is difficult to separate out gender, class and ethnicity in understanding discriminatory action.

Ethnic and racial identity

While racism and racialization are about the 'fixing' of a particular social identity onto a certain group, to its disadvantage, a focus away from the actions of the white majority considers the ways in which ethnic and racial identities may also be drawn upon in different ways by subordinated groups. Members of minority groups may actively use the perception of shared cultural attributes in creating and maintaining a collective identity, which may have a different meaning in different contexts and situations. For example, Asians in Britain may not self-identify themselves as 'black' in most situations and may in fact distance themselves from Caribbean groups. However, 'black' may be drawn on as a collective label in political struggles against oppressive practices of the 'white' majority. Ethnic or racial identities are not constant, therefore, but may be drawn on according to a particular identity's salience to a particular situation. This sense of ethnicity as 'cultural politics' or the 'politics of identity' stresses the active process by which ethnicity is given meaning and used strategically. An example of this, in the form of the introduction of 'cultural safety' in the education of health-care workers, is given later in this chapter.

Identities, however, are not just about collective action. There is increasing interest in the social sciences in the multistranded identities of people. The different strands will have greater salience in some social interactions than others. Take, as an example, a woman whose parents were born in India, who herself was born in England and who moved to Canada as a child. She has two young children from an arranged marriage and lives in an extended family household in a predominantly 'white' suburb. A fashionably dressed woman with a Western hairstyle, she works in a city office. She talks with her friends at work and in the neighbourhood about the latest films, music and city events but equally values the family gatherings and Indian cultural events, which she attends in her sari. She reads both 'mainstream' magazines and those published in the local Punjabi community, and a diverse selection of novels written by 'Western' and Indian writers. Each of these aspects of her life is blended in her self-identification and her social identity, but their importance, including that of her ethnicity, will vary according to whether she is at the neighbourhood preschool with her daughter, at the Sikh temple with other members of the Indo-Canadian community or in her workplace as a secretary in a large Canadian company. Such a person reflects the complexity of the task of understanding the organization of contemporary multicultural societies and the difficulties of analyses working with static categories that depict fixed ethnicities, stable cultures and a division of the world's people by race.

Activity 7.6

How would you describe your own cultural and ethnic background?

CULTURE, ETHNICITY AND 'RACE' IN OCCUPATIONAL THERAPY

The importance of culture as a framework for understanding and action applies to meanings and behaviours concerning health, illness and disability just as in other areas of life. It will influence how serious we think an illness is, the significance given to a particular disability and the actions we take in dealing with it. Occupational therapists have recognized the influence of culture on the meanings that occupations will have in people's lives, such as in the model of human occupation and the Canadian Model of Occupational Performance. Differences in the cultural background of practitioner and client are given primary focus in addressing difficulties in the therapeutic process, as in cases of communication problems and non-adherence (see Krefting & Krefting 1991 for an overview of the main themes addressed in occupational therapy). If we go beyond culture to consider the social construction of ethnicity and race, what sort of impact will this have on how we name and frame problems in occupational therapy? Both the culturalist and antiracist approaches that inform health service delivery and research models more generally hold implications for how the 'problem of culture' in occupational therapy can usefully be 'named and framed'.

CULTURAL OR ETHNIC SENSITIVITY

There is increasing recognition within occupational therapy that practitioners need to be aware of cultural issues. The understanding that people are cultural beings, guided by the shared values, meanings and knowledge of their culture as they respond to health problems, has dominated approaches addressing problems arising in cross-cultural clinical encounters. That is, the prob-lems encountered rest in differences in culturally shaped meanings and knowledge between the 'mainstream' practitioner and the culturally different client, and, as a corollary, resolutions will be found in addressing this cultural difference.

Explanatory model

Kleinman (1978) introduced the important concept of the explanatory model in applying anthropological insights to clinical practice. An explanatory model refers to the culturally shaped cluster of health beliefs and actions through which a person explains an illness and his or her expectations of what can or should be done about it. In the health-care encounter, patient and practitioner may be working with different and competing models. Each may hold different interpretations of a person's medical history, diagnosis, treatment expectations and ways of defining illness or disability as a problem. Such a mismatch may to lead to misunderstandings that result in ineffective treatment or non-compliance. The logical response to this problem is to negotiate this 'culture gap'. The practitioner will elicit the patient's explanatory model and then involve the patient in working out a treatment approach that is acceptable to both parties.

The explanatory model approach has considerable appeal. It is consistent with occupational therapy's client-centred practice and would appear to be sufficiently flexible to address the differences of explanatory models within broad cultural groupings, according to a client's age, gender and class positioning in society. Yet it tends to ignore the issue of power in clinical encounters and neglects the complexity of the relationship between action and behaviour, as in traditional functionalist approaches. Let us consider how these neglects may affect practice.

Power in clinical encounters

The doctor or therapist has power associated with his or her position in the medical system and holds authority as a result of the fact that biomedical knowledge is considered to provide the superior explanation of health problems. Its 'expert' status derives from its perceived objectivity, associated with the experimental method of science. Furthermore, while both lay and biomedical knowledge are cultural constructions, that of biomedicine is treated as somehow outside the cultural realm (Good 1994). Negotiation of explanatory models, then, is premised on the basis that biomedical interpretations are 'knowledge', cultural differences in explanation being subsumed as 'beliefs' in a hierarchy of medical knowledge. It may be difficult for the immigrant client to negotiate on equal terms when 'folk beliefs' are discounted as of little value and practitioners embody the power of science through their professional status. Constraints on negotiation may not be just a matter of individual communication between practitioner and client, but may also be built into the organization of health-care institutions and professional practice that reflect biomedical knowledge and ways of doing things. For example, ways of talking about and understanding illness through stories, as among some indigenous people, does not fit well with biomedically based assessments.

> Activity 7.7
>
> Can you think of any non-biomedical explanations of illness or health remedies that are common in your own cultural group?

The issue of power is dealt with indirectly in occupational therapy. It is acknowledged that occupational therapy, as a profession, embodies Western 'white' values, such as independence and the notion of requiring a balance between work, leisure and self-care for a healthy life, which may be of less importance to people of other cultures. Sensitivity to the norms, beliefs and values of other cultures is one way of averting any built-in ethnocentrism of occupational therapy models. In addition, a client-centred approach will alert the therapist to customary behaviours and valued occupations that can promote effective intervention rather than a reliance on therapeutic activities that reflect Western values. Occupational therapy also recog-

nizes that we, as well as our clients, are cultural beings and hold values and standards that shape our approaches to our work and our response to those we define as culturally different. Examination of our own core values and standards and our possible ethnocentrism is considered part of cultural sensitivity in practice.

Relationship between beliefs and action

The second neglect of the explanatory model, which spills over into all approaches relying on a concept of culture that emphasizes its learnt nature and internalization, is that of the complexity of linkages between ideas and behaviour. Studies show that beliefs and action do not necessarily enjoy a simple relationship as context always intervenes. Ideas about health, illness and appropriate health and illness behaviours are not fixed, as a fluid concept of culture would suggest. Studies show that 'new' knowledge can be incorporated into a person's cultural repertoire, while 'old' knowledge is reappraised as people share experiences, ideas and knowledge within the social networks of family, local community and work (Donovan 1986). Furthermore, a cultural repertoire may include both traditional and biomedical ways of dealing with ill-health that may be used concurrently without conflict from the patient's point of view. In addition, everyday circumstances may have as much effect, or more, on a person's ability to put into practice advocated management procedures than his or her explanatory model. Expediency in the context of everyday work demands, for example, may result in an older Chinese woman choosing to use painkillers instead of wearing a splint and using adaptive aids, rather than this resulting from a different explanation of the cause of rheumatoid arthritis or a cultural misunderstanding about its treatment (Dyck 1992). If a native client does not telephone to make or cancel an appointment, this may be because of a lack of a telephone and a difficult in reaching one rather than because of a lack of concern with time or an 'Indian way of doing things' (Waldram 1994).

When culture is viewed as the main determinant of what people do in a given situation, 'cultural characteristics' may be the first mode of explaining difficulties in the therapeutic process. Similarly to the way in which use of the concept of race by sociologists tends to reify it, so we come to a paradox in health care. If, in an attempt to be culturally sensitive when working with immigrant groups or indigenous peoples, we focus on culture, do we inadvertently 'blame' an individual and his or her culture for their health problems and ineffective treatment processes? This is a major concern for antiracist approaches suggesting that a culturalist stance, or ethnic sensitivity, plays a part in the racialization of minority groups.

ANTIRACIST APPROACHES

Proponents of an antiracist critique, such as Ahmad (1993), Stubbs (1993) and Sheldon & Parker (1992), note that, in a culturalist approach, the patient entering the majority health-care system tends to be the focus of the 'problem' because of his or her divergence from the majority culture rather than because of racism and processes of racialization. They see the conflation of culture, ethnicity and race as particularly invidious. The notion of culture tends to be simplified, and considered homogeneous, while the use of ethnicity and race as independent variables, rather than social and historical constructs, leads to their interpretation as objective determinants of behaviour. Following from this, most attention is paid to lifestyle, usually considered to be inferior, and cultural practices that are seen as contributing to health problems. The focus on individual cultural practices tends to ignore individual and institutional racism in health-care practice and health policy. It neglects the differential structural positioning of minority groups in society, which determines their access to a variety of material resources, including housing, employment and education, all of which influence people's health. If the power dimension of the construction of racialized social identities is ignored, the idea of 'natural' cultural characteristics promotes associations between certain

populations and particular health problems. For example, the high rates of diagnosis of British-born Afro-Caribbean Britons as schizophrenic and the notion of 'Asian rickets' feed an idea of 'impoverished cultures' without consideration of the ways in which conceptualizations of culture and race influence diagnostic interpretations (Ahmad 1993, Knowles 1991).

This way of thinking about cultural difference in health service delivery departs from an individual model of 'cross-cultural practice' to one more akin to the social model of disability. Just as the social and physical environment is interpreted as the cause of disability in the social model, so a parallel can be drawn with the antiracist perspective in that it is racism and social, economic and political processes of racialization that forge people's health and their access to effective health care. Moving away from a culturalist model implies that we must be wary of attributing all difficulties in the therapeutic process and 'unhealthy' lifestyles to culture and must consider the possibility that associations between particular health problems and certain groups may accompany entrenched inequalities arising from racism in society.

In occupational therapy, a consideration of socioeconomic conditions and inequalities arising from processes of racialization may lead to a different way of interpreting problems in practice, such as 'non-compliance', and a greater sensitivity to circumstances in clients' everyday lives that affect their priorities, shape the meaning that illness or disability has for them and may constrain their ability to adhere to occupational therapy interventions (Dyck 1995).

An antiracist perspective that focuses primarily on the structural positioning of subordinate groups in society sets up a convincing argument against an overreliance on culture in explanation. However, it is also subject to criticism. First of all, it is not easy to separate racism out in the explanation of particular groups' or individuals' health experiences. There are other oppressive relations, such as those of gender and class, that intertwine with racism and racialization. Like any reductionist argument, monocausal explanations disregard the complexity of social phenomena, including that of health and disability experience. Second, an individual's identification with a particular cultural or ethnic group can also provide positive experiences, for example in providing social and material support through a community's social networks. The extended family structure of some cultural groups may provide a setting in which the elderly may be cared for by family members in the home or a vibrant ethnic community can provide a sense of belonging in a climate of discrimination. Third, members of minority populations are not just passive 'victims' of racism but can organize collectively in furthering their health and health-care needs around a common cultural identification. This has occurred, for example, with regard to struggles over health care in New Zealand, where the concept of cultural safety in health service provision was launched. (See Jungersen 1992 for a discussion of the application of the concept in occupational therapy.)

CULTURAL SAFETY

The concept of cultural safety considers both structural inequalities in society and cultural differences in viewing health and health care. Rather than being concerned with improving health-care provision for immigrant populations, however, it was developed by a Maori nurse specifically for the purpose of bringing better health care to Maori people in Aotearoa/New Zealand. As with other subordinated native peoples, the health status of the Maori is poorer than that of the majority group, as measured by life expectancy, infant death rates and significantly different rates of certain illnesses. Their holistic concept of health, which includes the spiritual, the family, the mental and the physical, recognizes the importance of social and material conditions to health. The notion of cultural safety draws links between Maori health and their positioning within processes of historical and social change that have marginalized their culture and resulted in their social and material disadvantage. As a subordinated 'Other', their health and health-care knowledge are discounted

against the powerful biomedical paradigm. The focus of cultural safety and the structural subordination of Maori makes it a model directly applicable to other indigenous peoples who were colonized by white settlers, such as Aboriginal people in Australia, American Indians and the First Nations people of Canada.

The concept was first introduced in the context of nursing education in 1990 but has been adopted by other health professions, including occupational therapy. Cultural safety encompasses the idea that health workers are safe to practise with people from differing cultures. They need to be open-minded and flexible in their attitudes to consumers of their services and examine their own cultural realities and the attitudes they bring to their professional practice. Rather than a cursory knowledge of different cultural practices and beliefs, becoming culturally safe requires knowledge of the location of health problems within historical and social processes and exposure to alternative perspectives on health. In essence, it requires health-care providers to confront personal and structural racism. Although cultural safety was developed in the particular bicultural context of Aotearoa/New Zealand, its

---

Activity 7.8

Harminder, an Indo-Canadian woman, was admitted to an acute care psychiatric facility with a diagnosis of depression. She had a history of panic attacks, decreased appetite, low energy, chest pains and abdominal gas. She was confused about her admission to a psychiatric facility as she stressed the physical nature of her concerns, which her relatives attributed to the displeasure of her ancestors. Her treatment at the hospital consisted of counselling with a psychiatrist and occupational therapy group sessions. She blossomed in this miniature Canadian environment. When she was discharged from hospital, she had formulated many questions, the answers to which she believed would help her to avoid a recurrence of her illness. She wanted information about topics such as a healthy Canadian diet, her husband's drinking habits, childrearing and full-time work.

(Occupational therapy student case report)

How can sociological theories about multicultural society inform problem-solving in this client's situation? What types of information would you like to have more of in order to go beyond a 'culturalist' explanation?

principle of respect for different ways of 'seeing' and 'doing' health care and its recognition of the historical and social construction of a minority group's health status provides an approach that can be adapted to practice in multicultural societies.

CONCLUSION

Sociological analyses of cultural diversity in society indicate the complexity of issues of culture, ethnicity and race. What is 'cultural' in therapeutic relationships is not clear cut and is highly contextual. The value of fluid conceptions of culture and ethnicity is that they allow us to see the significance of culture to people in how they act in and interpret their social worlds, without seeing culture as deterministic or being 'fixed'. People may have deeply held values and ways of doing things that are of importance to them, but what these are cannot be assumed on the basis of our social identification of people as members of an ethnic or racial group.

Time may be a constraint in practice, but a narrative approach in problem-solving with clients is more conducive to working within the complexities of cultural difference than are assessments that make it difficult to relate the meaning of a health problem or disability to the context of a client's life. Similarly, in occupational therapy research, qualitative methods provide a means for people to define their reality rather than fitting data into a researcher's predefined categories.

Care must be taken in using ethnic or racial categories in clinical practice and research as their use in explaining behaviour further 'fixes' identity and makes assumptions about the 'cultural characteristics' of groups of people, which may lead to culture-blaming, to the neglect of the power differentials operating in society. Consideration of the structural positioning of subordinate groups in society also raises the question of the place of advocacy in occupational therapy. Is there room in our professional practice for combating institutional racism or advocating political change when we understand the effects on people's health of adverse social and economic conditions? The flexibility and open-mindedness of a cultural safety approach, with recognition of the effects of racialization on structural positioning and consequent access to resources, provides an important foundation from which to address the complex practice issues emerging in a context of multicultural society.

REFERENCES

Ahmad W I U (ed.) 1993 'Race' and health in contemporary Britain. Open University Press, Buckingham

Berger P L, Luckmann T 1967 The social construction of reality. Anchor Books, New York

Donovan J 1986 We don't buy sickness, it just comes: health, illness and health care in the lives of black people in London. Gower, Aldershot

Dyck I 1992 Managing chronic illness: an immigrant woman's acquisition and use of health care knowledge. American Journal of Occupational Therapy 46: 696–705

Dyck I 1995 Putting chronic illness 'in place'. Women immigrants' accounts of their health care. Geoforum 26: 247–260

Geertz C 1983 Local knowledge. Basic Books, New York

Glazer N, Moynihan D P 1963 Beyond the melting pot. MIT Press, Cambridge, MA

Good B J 1994 Medicine, rationality and experience. Cambridge University Press, Cambridge

Hannerz U 1992 Cultural complexity. Columbia University Press, New York

Jungersen K 1992 Culture, theory, and the practice of occupational therapy in New Zealand / Aotearoa. American Journal of Occupational Therapy 46: 745–750

Keesing R M 1987 Anthropology as interpretive quest. Current Anthropology 28: 161–176

Kleinman A 1978 Concepts and a model for the comparison of medical systems as cultural systems. Social Science and Medicine 12: 85–93

Knowles C 1991 Afro Caribbeans and schizophrenia: how does psychiatry deal with issues of race, culture and ethnicity? Journal of Social Policy 20: 173–190

Krefting L H, Krefting D V 1991 Cultural influences on performance. In: Christiansen C, Baum C (eds) Occupational therapy: overcoming performance deficits. Slack, Thorofare, NJ

Miles R 1989 Racism. Routledge, London

Miles R 1993 Racism after 'race relations'. Routledge, London

Porter J 1965 The vertical mosaic. Toronto University Press, Toronto

Rex J 1970 Race relations in sociological theory. Weidenfeld & Nicolson, London

Rex J 1986 Race and ethnicity. Open University Press, Milton Keynes

Sheldon T, Parker H 1992 The use of 'ethnicity' and 'race' in health research: a cautionary note. In: Ahmad W I U (ed.) The politics of 'race' and health. Race Relations Research Unit, University of Bradford/Bradford and Ilkley Community College, Bradford

Stubbs P 1993 'Ethnically sensitive' or 'anti-racist'? Models for health research and service delivery. In: Ahmad W I U (ed.) 'Race' and health in contemporary Britain. Open University Press, Buckingham

Waldram J B 1994 Cultural and socio-economic factors in the delivery of health care services to aboriginal peoples. In: Bolaria B S, Bolaria R (eds) Racial minorities, medicine and health. Fernwood Publishing, Halifax, Nova Scotia

8

The family

Christine Ravetz

INTRODUCING THE FAMILY

The family is an enduring social institution that is found in all societies throughout the world in one form or another. It can provide an environment conducive to physical and psychosocial development, but it can also be the source of much grief, both physical and psychological. Despite this, it remains a popular institution and one to which many wish to belong. The family unit is also the main source of care for people with mental illness, social stress and physical disability. For all these reasons, it is of concern to occupational therapists whose core interests are to assist their clients to live as they choose, both acknowledging and challenging the constraints of their own social environment. This chapter will assist in understanding this fundamental social entity.

TYPES OF FAMILY STRUCTURE

In spite of its apparently universal and familiar nature, the family is hard to define. This is because of its flexible and changing structure, which has continually altered. There is much interesting historical and anthropological literature on the family that highlights its variability with time and culture. However, in this chapter, we will focus on the family in modern Western societies.

A number of different types of family structure are dominant and easily recognizable. For example, the nuclear family structure and the extended family structure are very familiar

---

Box 8.1 Family structures

- The *nuclear family* consists of a husband, wife and their children living in one household
- The *extended family* consists of parents, children and close influential bilateral family kinship ties formed by the grandparents and aunts and uncles from both parental families

---

(Box 8.1). In many Western societies, there is arguably an idealized type of family, which is a husband and wife, living harmoniously together in one household with their small number of children – this has been called the 'cereal packet image' of the family (Haralambos & Holborn 1995).

Although this basic division between nuclear and extended family is helpful, it is perhaps oversimplified. Litwak (1960) identified the 'modified extended family' model. This recognizes the existence of the more or less self-contained nuclear family plus the importance of its links with the extended family, particularly grandparents. These links allow the exchange of significant services (such as financial loans or babysitting) between family members. Thus, although the members of the extended family may be separated by geography or by place of residence, they still behave in many ways as if they were living together. Wider car and telephone ownership facilitates this type of family structure. Other writers have produced variations on this theme. For example, Allan talks of the 'modified elementary family' (which has a more restricted network than Litwak's model and does not include uncles/ aunts, cousins, etc.). There is also Willmott's 'dispersed extended family', which is a network of supportive nuclear families who may have regular but not frequent contact with each other (Haralambos & Holborn 1995).

Defining the family

Giddens (1993, p. 384) defines the family as 'a group of persons directly linked by kin connections, the adult members of which assume responsibility for caring for children'. Note that he does not directly refer to marriage. Another definition, which refers to the contemporary custom of cohabitation, notes, 'A family is a married or cohabiting couple with or without children, or a lone parent with children' (Social Trends 1996, p. 53). This definition highlights the number of parents and children. The same definition also helps us to understand what a family is not. Social Trends (1996, p. 53) notes that 'People living alone are not normally considered a family.'

Activity 8.1

Make a poster that illustrates your family structure, indicating the nature of relationships and the places of residence. Compare your poster with those of others from your group.

Variations in family structures

There are many variations in families. Reconstituted families, for example, are units made up of couples who have been married before and bring the children of either or both previous marriages to the new family. The couple may also have children from their new union. Single-parent families are those in which one adult parent, who may or may not have been married, lives with his or her children without an adult partner in the household. Adults may choose to live together without children or may be unable to have children. Gay or lesbian couples may live together with the children of former heterosexual unions. In some cases, grandparents may raise children of their own children who may be dead or unable to accept the parenting role. We can thus conclude that the family is indeed a flexible and adaptable unit.

Activity 8.2

Would you accept the variations cited here as being 'real' families? Would most people accept them as real families?

Because of the changing nature of the family and its often predicted demise, it is useful to review some statistical evidence.

STATISTICS ON THE FAMILY

British statistical evidence illustrates the simultaneously stable and changing nature of the family. The figures below are taken from Social Trends (1995, 1996).

In 1991, in the UK, married couples with children or stepchildren constituted 71% of families. Four-fifths of dependent children live in a family with two parents. These figures indicate the stability of the conventional notion of a family of adult companionship, kinship, procreation and socialization.

Other patterns are apparent, however, and it is important to note that lone parents headed 22% of households, most lone parents being women. People are marrying later, on average at 26 for women and 28 for men. Women are having smaller families, the average number of children, for example, being 2.0 per family in 1970 and 1.8 in 1991, and are completing their families earlier. More women are choosing to remain childless. Divorce is more common, and in 1992 one divorce occurred for every two marriages that took place. Twenty-five per cent of divorces occur between the fifth and ninth year of marriage, and most are awarded to women because of male unreasonable behaviour. The stigma attached to divorce has declined, and people more readily consider divorce as an option within an unhappy marriage.

In spite of an overall decline in marriage rates and an increase in cohabitation patterns, marriage is still very popular: 90% of adults will marry at some time. Two-thirds of marriages are first-time marriages for both partners, but the number of remarriages has grown from 14% in 1961 to 34% in 1981. The average age for remarriage is 37 for women and 41 for men. At the other end of the scale, the number of teenage marriages has declined, but more babies are being born to teenagers who do not marry.

Activity 8.3

How many children do you have or would you like to have? Do you plan to marry? Do you agree that there is now less stigma attached to divorce?

In summary, people are cohabiting more often prior to marriage, marrying later, having fewer children, completing their families earlier, feeling easier about divorce and remarrying more frequently. Many families, however, adopt a conventional pattern. Once created, the family exhibits itself as a dynamic force and changes throughout its existence.

THE FAMILY LIFE CYCLE

Bond & Bond (1994) illustrate this dynamism by discussing the family life cycle. They divide the family cycle chronologically into childhood, youth, young adulthood, middle age and old age. Significant events can be identified from within this broad chronological plan:

- marriage or permanent partnership
- the birth of children
- children leaving home
- grandparenting
- the death of one spouse
- the death of the second spouse.

All of these events require major psychosocial readjustments. Involuntary deviance from the family life cycle or absence of the above events can also produce stresses and strains within the family. The inability to have children or the failure of children to leave home at the appropriate time, because of learning disability for example, may cause grief and a sense of failure. Disruption to the life cycle may also be caused by the early death of a spouse or child, or if both parents are killed, children may go to live with their grandparents.

Having looked at a dynamic element of the family, it is now time to look at an aspect that has stayed remarkably stable – the division of domestic labour.

DIVISION OF LABOUR IN THE FAMILY

The division of roles and tasks within the family remains surprisingly predictable. Delphy & Leonard (1992), writing from a feminist perspective, have highlighted how, despite changing patterns in employment, women still tend to spend twice as much time on domestic tasks as men. Pahl (1984), in his detailed study of the division of labour within the family, also indicated that women still tend to do the majority of household tasks. The study does indicate, however, that men share or help with many tasks, including childcare, shopping, cooking, and cleaning, but less so with washing and ironing. Many women now work, but the majority of men have higher and more consistent incomes. Men also organize repairs and household finance and discipline children more than women, although the sharing of duties and responsibilities does, of course, occur.

Activity 8.4

What is the division of labour in your household?

At this point, it is useful to review some of the different perspectives on the family, particularly some of the critical approaches.

PERSPECTIVES ON THE FAMILY

For much of the early part of the twentieth century, the family was an unquestioned institution, seen to be essential for the survival of society. This view was reflected in the work of functionalist sociologists. However, Marxists have historically taken a critical approach to the family, and more recently, feminists have drawn attention to the role of the family as a site of domestic violence. First, we shall deal with the functionalist perspective.

Functionalism and the family

The key functionalist sociologist Talcott Parsons believed that, although the modern family has lost some of its functions (the state for example, having largely taken over formal education), it is still essential to the maintenance of a stable society. Box 8.2 highlights the two tasks of the family – socialization and the stabilization of adult personalities – considered by Parsons to be essential in all societies (Haralambos & Holborn 1995).

Box 8.2 Parsons' essential family functions

Socialization: This process involves the internalization of a society's culture (its norms, values, etc.). The family is the main vehicle for this process in the early years of a person's life (hence the term 'primary socialization'), and, as the child grows up, other institutions (e.g. school) carry on the process (secondary socialization). Socialization not only involves the learning of behaviour, but also provides the context for the development of personality that reflects central social values (e.g. independence)

Stabilization of adult personalities: In adulthood, people are subject to all sorts of stresses and strains that could be damaging to their personalities. For functionalists, the family, in particular the relationship between husband and wife, provides emotional support and stability

---

The main criticisms of Parsons have centred on his focus on white, middle-class American families and his view of this form of family as an essentially good and necessary social institution. Marxists also see the family as functional, but functional to an exploitative capitalist society.

Marxism and the family

Karl Marx's collaborator, Engels, produced one of the earliest critical analyses of the family. In line with the general Marxist emphasis on economic determinism, Engels (1972) argued that the form that the family took was related to the economic system. Only where there is private (male) ownership of property do issues of paternity and inheritance become important, and it is in the monogamous nuclear family that these issues are addressed. For Marxists, the family is also seen as essential to capitalism, in that it is the place for the production of new workers and the maintenance of existing workers. Women maintain the workforce by performing many unpaid tasks such as cooking and cleaning. More recent Marxists, such as Zaretsky (1976), have focused on the family as a unit of consumption. Large numbers of isolated nuclear families mean a bigger market for consumer goods. Zaretsky also argues that the family is an important source of emotional support only because work is such an alienating experience in capitalist societies.

The Marxist analysis of the family shares elements with some feminist perspectives, for example the role of women in maintaining the workforce. For more radical feminists, however, the family serves not capitalism in particular but men in general. It is important to remember that there are a variety of feminist perspectives (see Chapter 6).

Feminism and the family

Earlier in this chapter, we highlighted the unequal division of domestic labour in the family, and below we will consider the unequal burden of caring that falls on women, but here, we will focus on the issue of domestic violence.

For many women, the family is anything but the nurturing place of stability that seems to emerge from the functionalist perspective. Some estimates identify violence against women by their male partners as accounting for over 70% of violence in the home and one in four of all violent crimes (Foreman & Dallos 1993). It is worth noting that, although violence seems to be more common in lower socioeconomic group households, men from all social classes are represented in the statistics.

Feminists have highlighted traditional notions of male authority – 'the head of the household', 'master in his own house' – which contrast with expectations of women to be nurturing, supportive and sensitive. Such ideas have supported a different response to violence in the home compared with violence between strangers outside the home. Domestic violence has been considered a private matter to be sorted out between those concerned. Women may also be faced with the response that they must have 'asked for it' in some way or at least have been partly responsible. Men, on the other hand, may be excused on the grounds of drink or stress.

The developing social response to domestic violence has been to treat the men concerned as pathological in some way and in need of therapy, or to treat them as criminals. A study in Minnesota, USA, looked at the rate of reoffending following different responses to domestic violence (Dobash & Dobash 1992). One-third of the men in the study were subject to mandatory arrest and detention; of these, 19% reoffended. In one-third of cases, couples were given 'advice', here the reoffending rate was 37%. In the final third of cases, the men were removed for a 'cooling-off period'; here the reoffending rate was 34%.

The question of punishment or therapy is a complex one. Responding with therapy *or* punishment alone seems inadequate: the former does not do enough to protect the victims, the latter does not aid understanding and therefore prevention (Foreman & Dallos 1993). Domestic violence is a complex and important topic, and we have only touched on a few issues here. Given the extent of the phenomenon it is quite possible that, as a therapist, one will come across the victims or perpetrators of domestic violence.

There are other critical perspectives on the family that we do not have space to consider here. For example, the psychiatrist R. D. Laing (Laing & Esterson 1970) is known for his work on family relationships and schizophrenia. Laing argued that manifestations of schizophrenia could be seen as reasonable within the context of family interactions. For Laing, the family is a destructive and unhealthy institution.

So far, the discussion has concentrated on issues relating to white families with a strong European identity. Yet in most Western societies in which occupational therapists practise, there is a wide range of ethnic diversity.

ETHNICITY AND THE FAMILY

Approximately 5.9% of the British population originate from a non-European culture. This proportion is growing and will probably stabilize at about 9% of the total population (Elliot 1996). Following the mass migrations from the Indian subcontinent, Africa and the Caribbean during the 1950s, 60s and 70s, the British population now consists of a sizeable proportion of people from ethnic minority backgrounds. Their religious backgrounds, class positions and cultural norms vary. Family structures similarly vary but have also demonstrated the same stability, flexibility and ability to change that families show universally. Elliot (1996), in her analysis of literature and research, has illustrated these differences and adaptations well.

For example, prior to migration, the dominant Afro-Caribbean family structure was of a single mother; it was matriarchal with strong kinship ties between mothers and daughters. This matriarchal family structure may have been the result of the tradition of African family relations, slavery (which made conjugal family relationships almost impossible) or socioeconomic conditions in the Caribbean, which made regular male work difficult to obtain. Trends indicate that, during the early days of migration to the UK, the family structure adapted and began to exhibit a pattern similar to that of the host culture. Recent studies, however, show that further adaptation has taken place, melding the different forms, and that the female-headed, single-parent family is still dominant.

Elliot (1996) also analyses the modifications that have occurred within Asian families. In spite of the differences in origin (India, Pakistan, Bangladesh and East Africa), religion (Islam, Hindu and Sikh) and class (either peasant or middle class, or based on the caste system), the traditional Asian family is characterized by the dominance of the male, patriarchal kinship line of grandfather, father and son and their spouses and unmarried daughters living in close proximity. The male members of the family control major decisions and finance, but the women control services within the family and exert influence from within. Family and community ties take precedence over individual plans or wishes, and marriage is based on family honour and compatibility rather than romantic love or individual choice. The family remains a constant source of support, sharing and communication. Younger people are often able to live in the parallel Asian and Western cultures or mix the two and are exerting more influence on decisions relating to them. Many, however, consciously and willingly adhere to traditional values and responsibilities (Elliot 1996).

As the nuclear family is an idealized model of a Western European family, so are the two family structures described above models of two types of families based on different cultural norms, values and socioeconomic influences found in Britain today. Ideal models should not be used to stereotype, but they do illustrate the richness and variety of family structures.

THE FAMILY AND THE FUTURE

If we accept that the family is flexible and changes over time while retaining constant recognizable characteristics, it is to be expected that the family will also change in the future. What can we expect? According to Gelles (1995), some adaptations that are becoming highly apparent include more flexible approaches to marriage, with higher divorce and remarriage rates, long periods of cohabitation prior to marriage, people marrying and having their first child at a later age, more overt long-term gay or lesbian relationships, possibly legalized in marriage at a future date, a continued decline in the birth rate, possibly to below replacement level, a continued increase in the number of single-parent families and changes to traditional roles as more women go out to work and more men become househusbands. Poverty is a major threat to the family. Gelles concludes that families are more diverse than they ever were and that, perhaps, 'the greatest strength of the family as a social institution is its ability to adapt and change in the face of social and cultural changes' (Gelles 1995, p. 511). The family will, it seems, remain as a major social institution.

THE FAMILY AND HEALTH

Of particular interest to occupational therapists is the family's relevance to health matters. The family is one of the most important social structures in which health is maintained. It provides health-enhancing structures and services such as a roof over one's head, a home, stability, relationships with people who give recognition and offer concern, a regular diet, stability, routine, regard, an identity, health care, hygiene, mutual support and social relationships (Gelles 1995). Even dysfunctional families provide some of these basic physical, social and emotional requirements for good health. In contrast, people living outside a family structure, for example single, divorced or widowed people, particularly men, tend to have higher mortality rates than those living within a family.

The family can also be a source of stress and illness, as highlighted by some of the critical perspectives discussed above. Some causes of stress are a lack of supportive partners, parental strife, poor childrearing patterns, poor parental health behaviours, a high incidence of violence, neglect and abuse, and perhaps above all, poverty. Numerous research studies have indicated the significant malfunctional role that the family has played in producing or exacerbating illnesses such as schizophrenia, depression, eating disorders, behavioural disorders, diabetes, cancer, heart disease, respiratory disorders and anxiety (McKenry & Price 1994).

Activity 8.5

How has your family influenced your health? Can you identify issues in any other families with whom you have had contact that have influenced the health of that family's members?

The family as a focus of care

The family is probably the most important health provider of any, far more so than statutory sources of care. The family is also a most important source of health promotion. Most short-term illnesses are managed within the family with relatively little medical intervention. Similarly, the family provides the most long-term and stable care in the case of chronic illness or disease (McKenry & Price 1994).

The onus of care, however, falls unevenly on family members. There appears to be a distinct gender difference in caring patterns, women being the most frequent carers. Responsibilities tend to fall on wives, mothers and daughters. The social consequences are that women will experience more frequent job or career interruptions, more interrupted sleep patterns, a reduction in leisure time, greater fatigue and more frequent minor illnesses, as is indicated by more frequent

visits to the general practitioner. Male carers tend to be retired and to look after one specific group: their wives (Bond & Bond 1994).

The demands on the family as main source of care have been increased by a number of recent social policy developments. The closure of large institutions, the reduction in the length of hospital stays and the development of community care policies have increased the number of vulnerable people living in the community, often with their families. The resources to offer proper support are not, however, always adequate, and it is often the family who bear the negative brunt of care, such as loss of income because of broken employment patterns and expenses relating to the disability. Social isolation can also occur, particularly if the disability involves socially unacceptable behaviour such as may occur as a result of schizophrenia or Alzheimer's disease. Other social factors contributing to pressure on the family as a caring unit are an increase in longevity, resulting in a greater number of infirm and vulnerable older people, particularly women, an increase in geographical mobility, which separates families, and larger numbers of working women and single parents.

Family involvement in health care

Families usually deal with short-term, acute illness or disease competently and with no permanent effects. Chronic problems, however, have long-term implications. Some of these prolonged implications are indicated in this section, which illustrates two specific examples of different types of situation dealt with by families, one relating to long-term mental illness and the other to long-term physical illness.

MacInnes (1996, p. 1) illustrates some of the difficulties encountered because of chronic mental illness. He states that 'people with schizophrenia are increasingly being supported when they leave hospital by relatives and informal carers'. Some of the identified problems experienced by families are lack of knowledge, social and leisure restrictions, financial difficulties and relatives' psychological ill-health.

Cambell (1994) indicates that many long-term

illnesses are directly related to poor family behaviour such as unhealthy eating habits, smoking and stressful relationships, which may be partially rectified through health promotion. He also plots the family response to serious physical illness. This follows a predictable course of a period of denial and disbelief, often followed by rapid mobilization of extended family resources and support, which then tend to decline over time as the chronic nature of the disability is realized. Some difficulty may be experienced in adapting to the long-term need dictated by the chronic illness. There is often a difficult period of renegotiation of roles and responsibilities, which fundamentally affects the notions of normal family life. Many families become closer, sometimes too close, thus affecting individual members' autonomy and independence. In other instances, the stress may result in family dysfunction, divorce or behavioural problems in children. The illness may begin to dominate family life. The family may become rigid, socially isolated and fearing change. However, it must be remembered that many families do adjust, seek out and are offered the correct amount of support, and reorganize their lives to incorporate the chronic illness.

This chapter has so far reviewed the sociology of the family and some, although by no means all, of the relationships between the family and health. There is a wealth of literature on both of these aspects of the family, and reading around the subject is encouraged. The discussion will now focus on the relevance of occupational therapy to the family.

OCCUPATIONAL THERAPY AND THE FAMILY

Both legislation and theoretical perspectives link occupational therapy and the family. Contemporary legislation in Britain, as Cassam (1995) discusses, has focused attention on community care and carers, which often means the family, as the main source of care for people with disabilities. The policy of community care, under-

pinned by a recognition that carers may require support from the statutory services, is well established in theory if not in practice and is unlikely to change. Occupational therapists play a key role in enabling community care, and will work with non-statutory carers, who are most likely to be family members.

In addition, there are theoretical approaches relevant to occupational therapy that support the inclusion of the family in treatment planning. The profession has a holistic perspective taking into account the many facets of the user's life. The perspective includes consideration of the biological problems linked to illness, disease and diagnosis, the psychological, emotional and cognitive aspects of human existence, including those relating to development and relationships, and the sociological considerations relating to the client's place within society. This holistic and biopsychosocial approach supports the notion that all aspects of the client's life must be considered as much as possible, including family relationships, particularly as the family is often so fundamental to client care.

Gitlin et al (1994) argue that an ethnographic framework assists the therapist in understanding the meaning and interpretation of events relating to disability from the family's perspective. Without this understanding, the intervention will be inoperable, as is illustrated in Case study 8.1.

Case study 8.1

Mrs Patel, a 70-year-old devout Muslim woman, developed a dense left hemiplegia. The occupational therapist, by talking to her family and applying an ethnographic framework, understood that the family accepted this as the will of Allah, that she would move into her son's home and that the family would take care of her. The therapist oriented her treatment towards assisting the family to cope and realized that many decisions would be made within the family, possibly even consulting the extended family in India. The therapist identified that a traditional rehabilitation model would not be appropriate in this case. The ethnographic approach can assist professionals in understanding the meaning of the illness from the client's perspective and therefore providing appropriate intervention.

LEVELS OF INTERVENTION

Contact between the therapist and the family will vary depending on different situations. Contact may be frequent, as in Case study 8.1, or minimal, as in Case study 8.2.

Case study 8.2

Ms Hepworth is a 46-year-old woman with a learning disability who now lives in a house with three other people. All four people had previously lived in a large institution for many years. Ms Hepworth has had minimum contact with her family for a long time and is not dependent on them either financially or emotionally. She has recently developed median carpal tunnel syndrome, and the occupational therapist has been working with her on activities of daily living. The therapist has had no contact at all with the family.

The relationship between people with learning disabilities and their families raises a number of issues. For many people, their families retain an influence over major life decisions well into adulthood. Consulting and informing families about decisions affecting their son/daughter or sister/brother is, of course, important. Indeed, there may in some cases be legal reasons for doing so. However, there may be conflict between an individual's desired lifestyle and what the family thinks is best for him or her. For this reason, self-advocacy and independent advocacy on an individual's behalf is seen as being increasingly important.

Activity 8.6

Identify other situations in which the therapist's involvement with the family will be high or low. If you had difficulty expressing your wishes, would you want your parents to have a major say in your life or would you choose someone else?

OCCUPATIONAL THERAPY AT DIFFERENT STAGES OF THE LIFE CYCLE

The family life cycle (Bond & Bond 1994), identified above, can be used to highlight different issues for occupational therapists working with families.

Childhood

Childhood disabilities may be congenital or acquired. In either situation, the family, particularly the parents, may experience disappointment and possible bereavement at the loss of their child's perceived potential. The therapist should be aware of and support their feelings. In the best multidisciplinary teams, family members are seen as part of the team alongside the occupational therapist and other professionals. Some therapists may work within family therapy units if behavioural or mental health disorders are apparent (Durant 1996). Others may work in specialist areas such as burns care (Church & Cooper 1996), as Case study 8.3 illustrates.

Case study 8.3

Four-year-old Lindsay pulled a hot drink off the table and sustained burns to her chest and right axilla. Her mother (a single parent supported by a sister who lives nearby and her divorced mother and partner) feels very guilty. The occupational therapist has made a pressure garment that must be worn 24 hours a day for the next 12 months. The mother assists the therapist in the fitting of the garment and has been instructed in its use and in Lindsay's skin care. In this case, the occupational therapist is also working with Lindsay's aunt and grandmother and her partner for the child's benefit. Intervention involves providing support, education and information, and has involved all the family in the specific therapy.

Youth

Adolescence is a time when people are usually still involved with their families but are becoming more independent. This is expected by both the parent(s) and the young person. If this normal pattern does not occur because of disability, and normal milestones, such as finding a job or going away to college, are not reached, the family, including the young person, may feel frustration, sadness and loss akin to bereavement. The occupational therapist may work with the family to normalize the pattern as much as possible to increase independence and ease the physical burden of working with a growing person, as Case study 8.4 illustrates.

Case study 8.4

Tony, who is 18 years old, has muscular dystrophy and has just finished his schooling. The family are all aware of his prognosis and wish to make the most of his future. The occupational therapist has been working with them all to advise on the design, funding and building of an extension to their house that will allow Tony more independence and make it easier for his family to care for his physical needs. However, at a recent meeting, Tony told his therapist that he would really like to live away from home but he does not know how to tell his parents that this is what he wants. Here, the therapist would be concerned with supporting Tony in his decision and looking into accessing funding to put together a package of care that might enable him to fulfil his ambition.

Young adulthood

During young adulthood, people normally leave the family and establish different roles in the wider social environment. Leisure and work activities, including establishing a career and travelling, are important. People may set up their own households, form longlasting partnerships and start new families. People's expectations of these newly established roles are often conventional and based on normal function as ascribed by dominant cultural beliefs. Long-term illness or disability disrupts these normal expectations and can cause stress and anxiety. People with disabilities experience higher unemployment and divorce rates, for example.

Activity 8.7

What do you want from your future? How would long-term illness or disability affect your plans? Consider the similarities and differences in how these plans would be affected if:

- you had schizophrenia
- you had rheumatoid arthritis
- your partner or children developed a chronic illness.

Case study 8.5 focuses on young adulthood. Occupational therapy is in this case focusing on family support and assisting Robert to establish a life away from his parents (MacInnes 1996).

Case study 8.5

Robert is 28 years old and has schizophrenia. He has spent some considerable time in hospital but for the most part lives with his parents, who have experienced a great deal of stress. His mother makes frequent visits to her doctor, and her husband has moved out of the family home. As part of the multidisciplinary team, which includes both parents, the occupational therapist has been involved with:

- the family support group, offering information and education on schizophrenia, coping strategies and the need for personal space and leisure
- running daily living skills groups at a day centre, the long-term aim being that Robert will live away from his immediate family.

Middle age

Middle age often involves more personal independence, greater financial security and increased social stability. Case study 8.6 involves a middle-aged women whose predicament has been made worse by her family situation.

Case study 8.6

Mrs Williams is aged 53 and lives in her own house with her adult son who bullies her and contributes little to the housekeeping. Her husband, always the dominant partner, died 2 years ago. Mrs Williams is known to the primary health-care team because of her long history of anxiety and depression. The occupational therapist helps Mrs Williams to access sessions on anxiety management, assertiveness skills and leisure activities at a community women's group. She also works individually with Mrs Williams to apply these activities to her particular needs. The mutually agreed aim is to help her to cope constructively with her son's behaviour and to create positive life experiences.

Old age

Old age is a time of major adjustment, sometimes made difficult by catastrophic events such as disabling illness and death. Case study 8.7 is illustrative of the events that may happen.

CONCLUSION

This chapter has offered a broad sociological analysis of the family, giving full recognition to

Case study 8.7

Mr and Mrs Ashworth are in their late seventies and live in their own home. Mrs Ashworth has Alzheimer's disease, and Mr Ashworth is her main carer. She is forgetful, agitated, restless, sometimes incontinent and occasionally a danger to herself. The team at the unit she attends include family support within their remit. The occupational therapist has been working with the couple at home. They have addressed safety issues and appropriate easy-to-manage clothing for Mrs Ashworth. The therapist, in general conversation, has been able to inform Mr Ashworth about the disease and the best way to work with his wife's abilities, as well as to discuss her disabilities. One result is that Mr Ashworth has initiated a series of short walks within a reasonable car drive from their home that expend his wife's residual energy and is making them both fitter. In this case, the therapist has worked with the family to support them in improving activities of daily living, safety, general health and quality of life.

the fluidity and adaptability of the family structure and its enduring characteristics. The role of the family in health matters and as a major health provision unit has also been explored. Illustrative case studies have been used to highlight some family situations that occupational therapists may find themselves dealing with, and the possible interventions that may be of benefit.

With the increasing deployment of occupational therapists in community settings, the family will become more and more integral to the therapist's caseload. The sociological literature highlights some of the tensions and questions raised by these developments, not least whether therapists are simply reinforcing and maintaining the role of women as the main providers of care. Therapists need to be aware of their own values and assumptions regarding who does the caring.

REFERENCES

Bond J, Bond S 1994 Sociology and health care. Churchill Livingstone, Edinburgh

Cambell T L 1994 Physical Illness in: Mckenry P C, Price S J (eds) Families and Change. Sage Publications, London

Cassam J 1995 The disabled person within the family and community. In: Bumphrey E E (ed.) Community practice. Prentice Hall, London

Church P M, Cooper R 1996 Burns. In: Turner A, Foster M, Johnson S E (eds) Occupational therapy and physical dysfunction. Churchill Livingstone, Edinburgh

Delphy C, Leonard D 1992 Familiar exploitation. Polity Press, Cambridge

Dobash R E, Dobash R P 1992 Women, violence and social change. Routledge, London

Durant B 1996 Family therapy. In: Willson M (ed.) Occupational therapy in short term psychiatry. Churchill Livingstone, Edinburgh

Elliot F R 1996 Gender, family and society. Macmillan, Basingstoke

Engels F 1972 The origin of the family, private property and the state. Lawrence & Wishart, London

Foreman S, Dallos R 1993 Domestic violence. In: Dallos R, McLaughlin E (eds) Social problems and the family. Sage, London

Gelles R J 1995 Contemporary families, a sociological view. Sage, Thousand Oaks, California

Giddens A 1993 Sociology, 2nd edn. Polity Press, Cambridge

Gitlin L N, Corcoran M, Leinmiller-Eckhardt S 1994 Understanding the family perspective: an ethnographic framework for providing occupational therapy in the home. American Journal of Occupational Therapy 49(8): 802–809

Haralambos M, Holborn M 1995 Sociology: themes and perspectives, 4th edn. Collins Educational, London

Laing R D, Esterson A 1970 Sanity, madness and the family. Penguin, London

Litwak E 1960 Occupational mobility and extended family cohesion. American Sociological Review 25

MacInnes D 1996 Relatives and carers of clients with schizophrenia. Mental Health Occupational Therapy 1(1): p. 1

McKenry P C, Price S H (eds) 1994 Families and change: coping with stressful events. Sage, Thousand Oaks, California

Pahl R E 1984 Divisions of labour. Basil Blackwell, Oxford

Social Trends 25 1995 HMSO, London

Social Trends 26 1996 HMSO, London

Zaretsky E 1976 Capitalism, the family and personal life. Pluto Press, London

9

Deviance

D. Jones

THE STUDY OF DEVIANCE

Human beings are a diverse species, and to a certain extent we celebrate that difference. Yet it seems that we can only tolerate so much diversity. Some forms of difference evoke a negative response, and no matter how non-judgmental we like to think we are, most of us will be able to think of some group or form of behaviour that consider decidedly odd, even going so far as to call it deviant.

> **Activity 9.1**
>
> Make a list of all those groups or behaviours you consider to be odd or deviant. Would most people agree with your list? What groups or behaviours might you expect to find on the average person's list that do not appear on yours?

As you have probably discovered from Activity 9.1, there is not necessarily a consensus about what constitutes deviance. A good measure of the extent to which something is considered deviant is the response to it in the form of negative legal *or* social sanctions. Sociologists have come to recognize this, and it is reflected in the scope of the literature. Clinard & Meier (1979, p. 15) note:

Deviance may thus take many forms far beyond the ones customarily alluded to by most people, for example, burglary, robbery, mental disorder, and prostitution. An almost endless variety of behaviours and characteristics are considered to be deviant by some people at least and encounter pronounced stigma in certain groups.

They go on to list, among other things, people with various disabilities, the 'obese', illegitimacy, the non-support of children and smoking marijuana.

Deviance, then, is a complicated issue. The answers to questions such as what counts as deviance and how it originates all depend on the theoretical perspective one takes. It is possible to identify three general approaches to deviance:

- the biological
- the psychological
- the sociological.

Although we are primarily concerned with the sociological approach, it is worth dealing with the other two as they may be encountered as explanations of deviant behaviour.

Remember, when reading this chapter, that the designation of something as deviant reflects the application of that label at some time and is not a judgment of the author.

BIOLOGICAL THEORIES

Biological theories tend to be concerned with the origins of deviance in individuals rather than with any issues around what constitutes deviant behaviour. For these theorists, people are predisposed to deviancy by their biological make-up. Two different types of biological theory can be identified:

- those claiming a link between body features and deviance
- those arising out of biomedicine.

Body features

The connection between body types and behaviour can be traced back as far as the ancient Greeks. However, more recent history has thrown up a number of theories of this type.

Phrenology and Lombroso

In the nineteenth century, Gall & Spurzeheim developed the science of phrenology; they believed that the mental capacities and tempera-

ment of an individual were reflected in the size and contours of the skull. This type of explanation declined in popularity but was given fresh impetus at the start of the twentieth century by Cesare Lombroso.

Lombroso believed, on the basis of his observations of physical characteristics and postmortem examinations, that deviants were in fact throwbacks to earlier stages of human development. He noted what he believed to be physical similarities between 'criminals, savages, and apes' (cited in Clinard & Meier 1975, p. 166).

Sheldon and body types

Another notable contribution to this group of theories came from W. H. Sheldon and his colleagues who identified three main body types, each with different personality traits (Box. 9.1). These body types were said to be related to the likelihood of occurrence of delinquent behaviour.

Box 9.1 Sheldon's body types (adapted from Levin 1988, p. 284–285)

- Endomorph – round puffy body/easy-going/relaxed
- Mesomorph – muscular/tough/angular/energetic/insensitive/assertive
- Ectomorph – slim/fragile/restrained/private/sensitive

Although these types of explanation are no longer given much scientific credibility, it is interesting to note the way in which they live on in the common imagination: we talk of people 'looking like' a criminal or a pervert.

Biomedicine

More recent biological explanations of certain types of deviance reflect developing biomedical knowledge. Deviant behaviour is, in this instance, considered to be the result of genetic or biochemical factors. Attempts have been made to uncover the genetic origins of particular forms of behaviour. In the mid 1960s, claims were made that the presence in some men of an extra Y chromosome (XYY syndrome) predisposed them towards antisocial behaviour (Suchar 1978, p. 61).

More recently a genetic predisposition towards alcoholism and homosexuality has been claimed. There has also been much interest in premenstrual syndrome and its effect on the behaviour of some women.

Activity 9.2

How far do you think biology can explain behaviour? Can you think of any recent cases covered in the media in which biological explanations of behaviour have been given or debated?

PSYCHOLOGICAL THEORIES

Some psychological theories of deviance cross over into a biological approach and others are far removed. As with biological theories, they tend to share the desire to find an answer to the rather limited question 'What type of individual does this sort of thing?' They are what Cohen (1966, p. 42) called 'kinds of people' theories. In this section, we shall concern ourselves with:

- a psychoanalytic approach
- personality trait approaches
- behavioural approaches.

A psychoanalytic approach

Psychoanalysis has undergone many developments and revisions since the acknowledged founder of the approach, Freud, laid out the basic concepts. Here, however, we shall deal only with classical Freudian theory.

Freud proposed that individuals are driven by primitive impulses, which are represented by the id. These impulses are brought under control by the super-ego, which represents the internalization of expected ways of behaving, as transmitted by the parents and other authority figures. The ego mediates between the wild pleasure-seeking id and the stern, controlling super-ego, enabling the individual to function on a day-to-day basis. In order to develop normally, people also have to progress through what Freud called the psychosexual stages of childhood (the oral, the anal and the phallic), the final stage being parti-

cularly important because of its association with the Oedipus complex.

For Freud, deviant behaviour occurs when there is an imbalance between the id, ego and super-ego, or when a person does not pass through the psychosexual stages or resolve the Oedipus complex. For example, unrestrained by an inadequate super-ego, a person may give in with wild abandon to the gratification-seeking id. Alternatively, an overdeveloped super-ego may drive a person to seek punishment, via the committing of deviant acts, for the feelings generated by the id.

For a more in-depth understanding of Freudian theory, the reader should consult an introductory text on the subject or any of the books written by Freud himself.

Personality trait approaches

One group of attempts to explain deviance focuses on the idea of personality 'traits' or characteristics. Here, it is assumed that personality is composed of generalized ways of acting based on an individual's combination of traits. Some authors, such as Hans Eysenck, suggest a biological basis for these traits, while others stress early childhood experience. All of these theories use some form of questionnaire to identify characteristics; for this reason, they have also been called psychometric approaches.

Eysenck produced a psychometric test, the answers to which he then related to two dimensions: introversion/extroversion and neuroticism/stability (Eysenck 1947). A third dimension, psychoticism, was later added (Eysenck & Eysenck 1976). Cattell (1950) also produced a psychometric test battery, the 16PF, which he related to 16 personality traits.

Using tests such as those developed by Eysenck and Cattell, researchers have attempted to discover the particular constellation of traits likely to be found in people displaying particular types of deviancy and to distinguish the deviant from the non-deviant. However, little evidence has been found to correlate personality traits with, for example, drug addiction or alcoholism (Clinard & Meier 1979, p. 111).

Behavioural approaches

When most people speak of behaviourism, they are referring to the set of ideas developed by B. F. Skinner. Skinnerian behaviourists suggest that an individual's actions are determined by the consequences resulting from that behaviour. Consequences are said to be positively or negatively reinforcing (Box 9.2), something being reinforcing if it increases the likelihood of that behaviour occurring again. It should be noted that reinforcement should not be confused with reward and punishment. A reward in the form of a sticky bun will only increase the likelihood of behaviour being repeated if the person has a sweet tooth. Similarly, those who went to school in the days of the strap and the cane will remember at least one individual upon whom this punishment had little effect.

Box 9.2   Reinforcement (based on Skinner 1953)

• *Positive reinforcement*: consequences that the individual likes and that therefore encourage repetition of that behaviour, for example praising a student for a seminar contribution in order to promote her contribution in future seminars. Token economy systems are based on positive reinforcement

• *Negative reinforcement*: consequences that the individual finds unpleasant, thereby encouraging behaviour that avoids those consequences, for example deducting marks for the late submission of assignments in order to get students to hand them in on time. Aversion therapy is based on negative reinforcement

---

It should be noted that it is not necessary to experience the consequence directly for it to be reinforcing. For example, a person who values money may continue to gamble simply because he or she knows of or has seen somebody else who has won.

The behavioural approach applied to deviancy suggests that such behaviours are a result of the reinforcement received for such actions. Self-mutilation could be positively reinforced by the provision of help from various health and social agencies where none was previously provided; the spoils from a successful burglary could be positively reinforcing for more burglaries. Bandura & Walters (1958, cited in Levin 1988, p. 286) explained violent delinquent behaviour in terms of the reinforcement received in the home; for example, parents would be observed achieving desired ends through violence.

The different psychological theories have been subject to much debate; behaviourists have been particularly critical of psychoanalysis, and they in turn have been accused of denying free will. Sociologists have pointed out the narrowness of individualistic psychological approaches and have drawn attention to the social context in which they operate. However, on another level, the sociological approach is not inherently better than a psychological one – its concerns are simply different.

Activity 9.3

Are you convinced by any of the explanations you have heard so far? What are their strengths and weaknesses?

SOCIOLOGICAL THEORIES

A sociological approach starts with the recognition that any form of behaviour occurs in and is constrained by the social setting in which it occurs. It is possible to discern identifiable patterns of behaviour even in what may seem like the most personal and individual of activities. From this starting point, many paths diverge, and in relation to deviance the paths we shall be exploring are:

• social pathology
• social disorganization
• anomie
• labelling (or societal reaction)
• varieties of deviance.

Social pathology

Much early sociological writing on deviance was only one step removed from individualistic approaches. Society was compared with an organism, and deviance was likened to a disease or 'pathology' affecting the health of the organism. For these theorists, the definition of deviance was not an issue; it was simply those behaviours which contravened the moral values of the very writers proposing the theory. As important as describing the phenomena being studied was a concern with social reform; for this reason, this approach is sometimes called a correctional one. Matza (1969, p. 20) highlights the West Side studies (conducted by the Russell Sage Foundation in 1914) as an example *par excellence* of the correctional perspective. He notes, 'A wholly dim view of slum life and of its close relation to diverse pathologies has been a staple of the correctional perspective, ... the slum was no less – and no more – than a pathological growth in modern society.'

Although by the 1930s this approach was disappearing within sociology, the notion of certain behaviours being a sickness afflicting society lives on.

Social disorganization

As the social pathology perspective was declining in popularity, so there emerged a group of theorists based at the University of Chicago who developed an ecological or demographic approach. They became known as the Chicago School, and included people such as Robert Park, William Thomas and Florian Znaniecki. This School was more interested in developing theoretical explanations of deviance than in social reform.

The typical Chicago approach involved using statistics provided by various legal, social and health agencies to create social maps of the urban environment. These maps indicated what Park called the 'moral regions' of the city (Park et al 1925). An area called the zone of transition, which surrounded the central business core of the city, was identified. In this zone were to be found the highest rates of crime, prostitution, alcoholism, etc. This area was also characterized by high levels of social disorganization: transient populations, unstable social networks and poor housing. The result was an area in which deviant and non-conformist behaviour was tolerated, an area, as Park put it, 'in which a divergent moral code prevails' (Park et al 1925, p. 45).

However, it was not just in particular neighbourhoods that deviance was to be found. The effect of loose social restraints was illustrated by Hayner (cited in Matza 1969, p. 46). In relation to 'temporary' deviance, he noted:

Released from the bonds of restraint operative in smaller and more intimate circles, the individual tends to act in accordance with his impulses rather than after the pattern of ideals and standards of his group. Among heavy offenders for stealing hotel property are listed men and women who in their own communities command respect, but on going into a hotel, take a moral holiday.

The causes of deviation for the Chicago School lay not in individuals but in the nature of the disorganized social environment in which they lived. It is interesting to note how the popularity of this view lives on in the notion of lack of 'community spirit' being implicated in the problems of inner-city areas.

Although the ecological approach represented a significant advance in many respects, it also suffered a number of flaws. One major criticism related to the use of official statistics, which at best only recorded *identified*, rather than actual, rates of deviance. Nor did the studies take into consideration the role of various agencies in determining who ended up in the statistics. As Suchar noted, 'Juveniles of *all* social classes and in all areas commit delinquent acts, but only some get caught and get their names placed in juvenile court records' (Suchar 1978, p. 81). Other criticisms related to a failure to deal with issues such as white-collar crime and to explaining why only some of those living in a disorganized social setting became deviant.

Anomie

Around the same time that the Chicago School were carrying out their studies, there emerged one of the most influential perspectives on deviance. This approach that had its origins in the functionalism of Durkheim and was associated with the structural functionalism of Talcott Parsons. A key concern here is the strength, or lack of strength, of social norms.

Although Durkheim and the structural

functionalists, like the social pathologists, used an organic analogy, it was a much more sophisticated model. For Durkheim, social pathology was, to a certain extent, relative, normal and even useful (Suchar 1978, p. 22). His classic study *Suicide* could be said to be one of the first attempts at the sociological analysis of deviant behaviour. In this study, Durkheim proposed that there were four types of suicide, each related to the existing social organization and level of social integration (Box 9.3).

Box 9.3 Durkheim's types of suicide

Egoistic	Occurs where there is strong emphasis on individualism and few social ties
Altruistic	Occurs where there is high level of social organization, suicide being expected in certain circumstances
Fatalistic	Occurs as a response to an intolerably oppressive situation, for example slavery
Anomic	Occurs where there is a state of normlessness, where there are no clear guidelines on behaviour or expectations

---

Box 9.4 Merton's (1938) types of deviance

Conformity	Person accepts valued goals and uses accepted ways of achieving them. Non-deviant
Innovation	Person accepts culturally valued goals but, in the absence of legitimate opportunities to achieve them, turns to alternative means, for example theft to gain money and gang membership to gain prestige
Ritualism	Person overidentifies with culturally accepted means of achieving valued goals, perhaps becoming a 'workaholic' or obsessional and bureaucratic
Retreatism	In the face of an inability to obtain the desired goals, the person gives up on both the goals and the means of achieving them. Retreatism may present as mental health problems or withdrawal into a world of chronic drug and alcohol abuse
Rebellion	Person consciously rejects both goals and the means of obtaining them. They may, for example, choose to live in some form of alternative community or join a radical political group

---

The idea of a collapse in the norms guiding behaviour, a state of anomie, was taken up and developed by R. K. Merton, who applied the concept to deviant behaviour in general. Merton's proposition was that 'social structures exert a definite pressure upon certain persons in society to engage in non-conforming rather than conforming conduct' (Merton 1957). Merton proposed that where there is a gap between certain culturally valued goals (money, education, consumer goods, etc.) and the legitimate means available for achieving those goals, individuals may respond in different ways (Box 9.4).

For Merton, innovatory deviance in particular was most likely to occur in the lower socio-economic classes because of restricted access to legitimate means of obtaining valued goals,

---

Activity 9.4

Refer back to your list of deviant behaviour. In which of Merton's categories would you place the behaviour recorded?

---

owing to unemployment, low pay, etc. Note that, for Merton, deviance is not 'abnormal' but is in fact an understandable adaptation on the part of individuals to social pressures.

Merton recognized that innovatory deviance was not peculiar to the lower classes and that official statistics on, for example, crime could not be taken at face value. Despite this, he has been criticized for failing to explore in sufficient detail deviance among the middle and upper classes. Merton's analysis also fails to account for people who achieve valued goals through legitimate means *and* engage in deviant behaviour – professional people who use drugs on a 'recreational' basis, the politician who visits a prostitute to be dominated. Lemert (1964) criticized anomie theory for its inability to account for the exclusion experienced by people with disabilities. In this case, it is deviant status that limits their access to legitimate means of achieving valued goals; thus deviance precedes rather than follows a lack of opportunity.

A broader criticism of Merton relates to his

structural functionalist background. Structural functionalism has been criticized for 'reifying' society (Jones 1993, p. 40). This means that society is treated as an independent 'thing' rather than being something socially constructed by its members and powerful groups. Structural functionalists fail to deal adequately with the question of where valued goals originate or why individuals accept or reject them.

Labelling theory

One of the most influential theories about deviance, which has had an impact beyond its popularity within sociological circles, is labelling (or societal reaction) theory. Labelling theory, unlike the perspectives so far, falls within the interactionist, antipositivist approach within sociology. It is important to note that labelling theorists do not form a unified school of thought. Indeed, Edwin Lemert, who provided many of the initial key concepts, was critical of other writers (such as Howard Becker) associated with the perspective (Lemert 1972, p. 16). For labelling theorists, important issues are the process by which behaviour comes to be labelled as deviant, who does the labelling and the consequences for the individual so labelled.

The classic labelling theory definition of deviance was provided by Becker, who stated (cited in Scott & Douglas 1972, p. 40):

deviance is *not* a quality of the act the person commits, but rather a consequence of the application by others of rules and sanctions to an offender. The deviant is one to whom the label has successfully been applied; deviant behaviour is behaviour that people so label.

Labelling theorists, more than most, emphasized the cultural and situational relativity of deviant behaviour. Thus taking another's life is not considered to be deviant if it occurs on the wartime battlefield, nudity in public is the norm on some European beaches, and cocaine was once legal and widely used.

If any behaviour is not inherently deviant, how do we explain how something comes to be deviant? The answer for most labelling theorists is that certain groups in society (e.g. the police,

the medical profession and the government) have the power and the means of control available to them to define what is and what is not deviant. Becker used the term 'moral entrepreneurs' to refer to those in a position to influence the designation of certain acts as deviant. Such groups are able to manipulate the media and politicians to respond to problems about which 'something should be done'. For example, single parents and absent fathers have been subject to much attention in Britain, and Christian fundamentalist groups in the US have turned their attention to the lyrics of rock music.

Activity 9.5

Can you think of any recent campaigns to 'get something done' about certain acts or groups of people? Who was making the demands, and what is the history of the behaviour or group targeted?

Lemert, who originally introduced the notion of societal reaction being involved in the creation of deviance (Lemert 1951), also distinguished between two types of deviance: primary and secondary. Primary deviance is behaviour that may or may not be recognized as undesirable but in either case does not attract serious sanctions or have major implications for individuals in terms of their view of themselves. Secondary deviance refers to behaviour that has attracted a societal reaction in the form of the application of some form of label (criminal, sexual pervert, alcoholic, etc.) and sanctions such as isolation or a restriction of opportunities. Lemert (1972, p. 48) notes, 'the original "causes" of the deviation then recede and give way to the central importance of the disapproving, degradational and isolating reactions of society'. The label becomes a 'master status' to which people respond, ignoring all other non-deviant aspects of the individual. Those so labelled then undergo a process of internalization by which they come to incorporate the label and its associated expectations as part of their self-identity; in Lemert's terms, they adopt a 'deviant identity'.

Another distinction made within labelling theory is between ascribed and achieved deviance.

In the case of ascribed deviance, the label is applied following the observation of some characteristic over which an individual has little control (e.g. physical impairment). Achieved deviance refers to the application of a label following observation or knowledge of some behaviour.

Stigma

The notion of stigma is one which often appears in the writing of labelling theorists, the concept being associated with the American sociologist, Erving Goffman. The word 'stigma' is used to refer to a sign or mark that discredits a person in the eyes of others. The stigma can be obvious, for example physical disfigurement, or hidden, as in the case of a criminal record. Goffman was interested in the ways in which stigmatized individuals manage their interactions with others, i.e. how they deal with the fact that others consider them to be in some way of less value.

Labelling theorists have done much to enrich the study of deviance and firmly establish the notion of the relativity of deviance and the role of powerful groups in determining who gets labelled. However, the perspective has also been subject to criticism. Although labelling falls within the interactionist perspective, it has been criticized for not being sufficiently phenomenological (Warren & Johnson 1972, p. 69–92), i.e. it fails to examine the meaning that deviants attach to their own behaviour. As Bilton et al (1981, p. 601) note, 'the *degree of choice* and *consciousness* of actors, and the *meaning* of their behaviour to them, is apparently devalued by the labelling perspective'. The gay community is a good example of a group of people who do not create a 'deviant self-identity' for themselves. That is to say, they construct a positive self-identity – hence 'gay pride'. Labelling theory has also been criticized for overstating the issue of relativity as certain behaviours, incest for example, are almost universally considered to be deviant, although it is true that different incestual relationships are taboo in different societies. The theory has been accused of romanticizing deviance by focusing on what have been called 'marginal' or 'exotic' forms of deviance (Bilton et al 1981, p. 600) and ignoring activity such as rape and violent crime.

Varieties of deviance

One approach that recognizes and deals with the issue of varieties of deviance is that proposed by Hagan (see Abercrombie et al 1994, p. 476). In recognition of the fact that there is a clear difference between glue-sniffing and serial murder, he suggests that variations from social norms can be placed on a continuum of seriousness within a framework constructed of three dimensions (Box 9.5). In the case of consensus crimes, for example rape, there would be high agreement about the wrongfulness of the act and a severe social response, and the act would be evaluated as very harmful. In the case of social diversion, for example punk rock, there would be little agreement about wrongfulness, the social response would be mild and the deviation would be considered relatively harmless.

This perspective provides a useful approach to the description and classification of deviant acts, and it can also be used to chart the ascent of deviance from social diversion to, for example, conflict and crime – or vice versa. Some would argue that smoking, for example, is moving from being a social diversion to a social deviation. On its own, this approach is, however, insufficient. We need to look to other theories to provide

---

Box 9.5 Varieties of deviance: dimensions and types

Dimensions of seriousness
- Social agreement about the wrongfulness of the act
- Social response elicited by the act
- Social evaluation of the harm elicited by the act

Types of variation
- Consensus crimes – result in public outcry, for example child abuse or mass murder
- Conflict crimes – subject to some divided opinion, for example squatting and civil disobedience
- Social deviations – negatively viewed but are not criminal, for example schizophrenia and transvestism
- Social diversions – mildly disapproved by some sections of the population, for example style of dress, language or lifestyle

more in-depth explanations of the origins of deviant behaviour and the process involved in its designation and reaction to it.

DEVIANCE AND OCCUPATIONAL THERAPY

If we accept the notion of deviance as incorporating all those behaviours or characteristics subject to legal or social sanction, it is clear that occupational therapists come into contact with such people on a day-to-day basis. Therapists will have as their clients people who, because of their diagnosis (schizophrenia, learning disability, cerebral palsy, etc.), or because of some aspect unrelated to their referral (homosexuality, being a new-age traveller, etc.), are stigmatized. Being aware of the impact that this has on people is important if, in planning therapeutic interventions, we are to take into account social as well as biological and psychological factors. For this reason alone, occupational therapists should be interested in the study of deviance. However, the literature also merits study because it can throw light on others' views of 'odd' or 'different' behaviour. In the rest of this chapter, we will briefly consider this issue, but we will pay particular attention to the way in which sociological theories, primarily labelling theory, have had a direct impact on the provision of services, therapeutic interventions and the politics of disability.

EXPLAINING DEVIANCE

As a student and as a practising therapist, you will hear many different reasons given by carers and other professionals for what may be called deviant behaviour. Being aware of what sociologists have written about deviance can help in reflecting on one's own and others' under-standing of deviance. It is possible to discern in people's explanation of deviance echoes of earlier biological, psychological or sociological theories. For example:

'I wouldn't be surprised, I always thought he looked a bit odd a bit odd you know.' (biological/genetic explanation)

'Take no notice, it's just the type of person she is.' (personality trait explanation)

'It's understandable really given his social circumstances.' (anomie or social disorganization)

'You won't get her to do dressing practice; she's adopted the sick role.' (labelling theory)

This final example is an interesting one as the term 'sick role' (see Chapter 5) is a sociological concept commonly used by health professionals who have had a little exposure to the discipline, possibly only through a basic course. The danger is that, without proper understanding of the concept, it can be misused and misapplied. From the perspective of labelling theory, one could see the term 'sick role' as being no more than another label applied to an individual, resulting in a negative response. The person may well have adopted the sick role, but there may also be other explanations for the behaviour, which should be explored.

A study by Rosenhan (1980) provides a good example of the care required in interpreting behaviour on the basis of a label. Rosenhan claimed to demonstrate how normal behaviour can be interpreted as deviant. In his study, he had a group of people admitted to a psychiatric unit by instructing them to show symptoms of schizophrenia. Once admitted to hospital, they were advised to behave perfectly normally. Interestingly, the behaviour of the 'pseudo-patients' was described by staff in psychiatric terms. For example, one person when found pacing the corridors was asked if he was 'nervous'; 'No, bored', was his response. Other pseudo-patients observed taking notes were described as 'engaging in writing behaviour'.

LABELLING AND NORMALIZATION

The principle of normalization (latterly called social role valorization), as developed by Wolfensberger (1972, 1984), has had a major impact on services to people with learning disabilities, particularly in the USA and UK. Many service providers for this client group advertise the fact that normalization principles guide what they do. As Emerson (1992, p. 6) points out, Wolfensberger based his ideas explicitly on the work of labelling theorists. The principle of normalization proposes that labels such as mental handicap/retardation, etc. cause individuals to be cast in the role of deviant and their behaviour, and the response of others to them, to be determined by expectations surrounding those labels. In order to reduce the effect of these labels, Wolfensberger developed a strategy that placed an emphasis on:

1. reducing elements that made individuals stand out (special buses, housing, etc., and congregating people together in large groups)
2. aiming to give people valued social roles to counteract negative perceptions (examples of valued roles being friend, neighbour, student, etc.).

Normalization has, to a certain extent, been overtaken by other philosophies (e.g. O'Brien and Lyle's (1989) five service accomplishments), which, despite having their roots in Wolfensberger's work, are also different in many respects. Just as labelling theory was criticized for failing to take sufficient account of the perspective of those being labelled, so has normalization been taken to task for failing to value individuals as individuals. That is to say, normalization sets out to change what appears different about individuals rather than to change people's response to that difference. More recent approaches to learning disability reflect a concern with valuing diversity and participation. This change in emphasis suggests that a shift in therapeutic intervention is required. While it is still valid to reduce practices that mark people out as being different, it is equally important to gain acceptance of people in their own right through their participation, with the support required, in everyday life.

LABELLING AND THE POLITICS OF DISABILITY

The idea that the various labels applied to disabled people are an important part of the discrimination they experience is an important issue in the politics of disability. Although Goffman himself has been criticized for the way in which he talks about disability (Abberley 1993, p. 110), the influence of labelling theorists is clear. It is possible to discern a two-pronged approach to the use of labels. The first is concerned with trying to combat the effect of a diagnostic label attaining the level of a master status. This is reflected in the demands of some activists that they are more than their disability and that the term 'person with a disability' rather than 'disabled person' should be used (Hasler 1993, p. 281). Others have argued for the use of such terms as 'differently abled' or 'physically challenged'. Some therapists have taken up this notion and will avoid phrases such as, 'He's a hemi.', 'She's a stroke' or 'He's a CP' and tend to refer to people as clients rather than patients. This approach is also reflected in the move away from terms that are seen as being negative, for example 'geriatric' or 'mental handicap/retardation', and

---

Case study 9.1 Labelling in practice

I remember the Team having this big debate about whether we should change our name from 'Community Mental Handicap Team' to 'Community Team for People With Learning Disabilities'. I didn't realize it would arouse such passion! On the one hand I couldn't understand the opposition; after all, we changed from using terms like 'idiot' and 'imbecile' in the past. On the other hand, for some of the team members, I felt that they preferred the term 'mental handicap' precisely because they saw our clients as being essentially different from us and agreed with the general public's ideas about mental handicap.

(Occupational therapist working in learning disability services)

the designation of services as being for 'mental health' rather than 'mental illness'. Some therapists will read only the minimum information necessary from case notes in order to avoid being unduly influenced by the contents and any negative labels contained therein. All of these examples can be seen as attempts to replace or avoid labels that are seen as evoking a negative reaction.

The second approach to the issue of language perhaps reflects those who criticized labelling theorists for failing to take into account the ability of actors to apply their own meanings to labels. The concern here is to redefine or subvert the meaning of labels. Hasler (1993, p. 281) notes of some disability activists that '[They] took words used by the World Health Organisation … and redefined them saying that disability was not the lack of function … but was the social response to that lack of function'. Thus people with physical or cognitive impairments are indeed 'disabled people': they are disabled by society.

It is unfortunate that the issue of the labels used to refer to people has been 'hyped up' and clouded by popular press polemics against 'politically correct' language. If, however, our profession is serious about being client centred, how our clients prefer to be referred to is an important issue.

CONCLUSION

The study of the sociology of deviance has hopefully been shown to be of importance to occupational therapists. Not only can study of this area help to develop awareness of one's own and others' explanations of behaviour, but it can also put into context the development of philosophies such as normalization that have had an impact on service provision and therapeutic intervention. The use and abuse of labels has also been an important issue among people with disabilities and their concern to develop a social model of disability. This particular topic is explored in more detail in Chapter 15.

REFERENCES

Abberley P 1993 Disabled people and 'Normality' In: Swain J, Finklestein V, French S, Oliver M (eds) Disabling barriers – enabling environments. Sage, London

Abercrombie N, Warde A, Soothill K, Curry J, Walby S 1994 Contemporary British society. Polity Press, Cambridge

Bilton T, Bonnett K, Jones P, Stanworth M, Sheard K, Webster A 1981 Introductory sociology. Macmillan, London

Cattell R B 1950 Personality: a systematic theoretical and factual study. McGraw-Hill, New York

Clinard M B, Meier R F 1979 Sociology of deviant behaviour, 5th edn. Holt, Rinehart & Winston, New York

Cohen A K 1966 Deviance and control. Prentice Hall, Englewood Cliffs, N J

Emerson E 1992 What is normalisation? In: Brown H, Smith H (eds) Normalisation: the reader for the 90's. Routledge, London

Eysenck H J 1947 Dimensions of personality. Routledge, London

Eysenck H J, Eysenck S B G 1976 Psychoticism as a dimension of personality. Hodder & Stoughton, London

Hasler F 1993 Developments in the disabled people's movement. In: Swain J, Finklestein V, French S, Oliver M (eds) Disabling barriers – enabling environments. Sage, London

Jones P 1993 Studying society: sociological theories and research practices. Collins, London

Lemert E M 1951 Social pathology: a systematic approach to sociopathic behaviour. Prentice Hall, NJ

Lemert E M 1964 Social structure, social control and deviation. In: Clinard M B (ed.) Anomie and deviant behaviour. Free Press, New York

Lemert E M 1972 Human deviance, social problems and social control. Prentice Hall, Englewood Cliffs, NJ

Levin W C 1988 Sociological ideas, 2nd edn. Wadsworth, Belmont, CA

Matza D 1969 Becoming deviant. Prentice Hall, Englewood Cliffs, NJ

Merton R K 1938 Social structure and anomie. American Sociological Review 3: 676

Merton R K 1957 Social theory and social structure. Free Press, Illinois

O'Brien J, Lyle C 1989 Framework for accomplishment. Responsive Systems Associates, Atlanta, GA

Park R E, Burgess E W, Mckenzie R D 1925 The city. Univ of Chicago Press, Chicago

Rosenhan D L 1980 On being sane in insane places. In: Mechanic D (ed.) Readings in medical sociology. Free Press, New York

Scott R A, Douglas J D (eds) 1972 Theoretical perspectives on deviance. Basic Books, New York

Skinner B F 1953 Science and human behavior Macmillan, New York

Suchar C S 1978 Social deviance: perspectives and prospects. Holt, Rinehart & Winston, New York

Warren C A B, Johnson J M 1972 A critique of labelling theory from a phenomenological perspective. In: Scott R A, Douglas J D (eds) Theoretical perspectives on deviance. Basic Books, New York

Wolfensberger W 1972 The principle of normalisation in human services. National Institute on Mental Retardation, Toronto

Wolfensberger W 1984 A reconceptualisation of normalisation as social role valorisation. Mental Retardation (Canadian) 34: 22–25

10

Health and illness

R. K. Jones   D. Jones

SOCIOLOGY OF HEALTH AND ILLNESS

The beginnings of medical sociology (or the sociology of health and illness as it is now called in the UK and other Commonwealth countries) emerged at the end of the nineteenth and early twentieth centuries and was known as social medicine. It was mostly concerned with medical institutions and what happened in those institutions. Medical sociology generally dealt with the application and use of sociological concepts and methods to facilitate the work of the medical profession. Over the past 20 years, broader issues have emerged that concern themselves with the entire repertoire of forces that influence the well-being of individuals in society. These issues include not only historical dimensions and how different periods have 'seen' or thought of 'the body', but also an analysis of the biomedical model, which dominates Western medicine and the health beliefs and practices we hold about the body (the social construction of ideas about the body). In addition, the nature of power and the professions is a dominant concern.

Many of the chapters in this book deal with issues from the field of the sociology of health and illness. For example, Chapter 12 includes detail on the power of professionals, and Chapter 5 deals with the concept of the sick role. This chapter will focus on models of health and the nature of medical encounters (what happens between health-care staff and their clients). We will also explore the impact of chronic illness on the individual, particularly in terms of self-identity. These issues clearly raise interesting questions for occupational therapists about their interactions with clients and how those clients view themselves at different stages of their illnesses.

A SOCIOLOGICAL APPROACH TO HEALTH AND ILLNESS

A sociological approach to knowledge about health and illness differs from the biomedical approach in that it does not assume the objective existence of what medicine categorizes as disease (Freund & McGuire 1995). Social constructionism, mentioned elsewhere in this book, plays a key role in the way in which sociologists have approached this subject.

Activity 10.1

Revise your understanding of the term 'social constructionism'.

The sociologist does not take for granted that disease entities exist in nature and await 'discovery'. Social constructionism does not *necessarily* call into question the reality of disease or illness states or bodily experiences. Thus it is acknowledged that people do experience real pain, sickness and death. However, this approach emphasizes that these states and experiences are known and interpreted through social activity and can therefore be examined using cultural and social analysis (Lupton 1994).

In highlighting the social construction of health and illness, it can appear as if biology is being ignored, and some sociologists have been critical of the apparent absence of the body in the literature. In the same way that traditional medical approaches seem to ignore the link between the mind and the body, so some sociologists seem overly concerned with the social, forgetting that we inhabit a physical entity. As Bendelow & Williams (1995, p. 140) put it, it can seem at times that the body is reduced to 'a discursive construct'. It is thus important to remember that we have a body, a physical entity, that occupies space, and when we die it will continue to exist (until it rots away). At the same time, however, we also experience our bodies, and that experience is mediated by social and cultural influences.

Our bodies do not often impinge on our consciousness until they start to go wrong or change in some way. For example, most of us tend not to be aware of our hearts beating. However, when we do become aware of this (perhaps because of an increase in rate), we not only have the physical sensation, but also begin to attach meaning to possible causes of our awareness – are we ill, in love, unfit or getting old? The physical experience has a personal, social and cultural meaning. We will return to these issues when we consider the impact of chronic illness on self-identity. Before doing so, we need to examine the different models of health and illness.

MODELS OF HEALTH AND ILLNESS

Although other models do exist, such as the folk or traditional healer model (mostly found in Africa) and the harmony or balance model (in Asiatic cultures), it has been customary to divide the history of Western medicine into three stages (Box 10.1).

Despite the increasing acceptance of alternative therapies, such as acupuncture, by doctors, it is still true to say that the biomedical model has an enduring influence on the way in which we view health and illness.

Box 10.1 Western models of health and illness

- *Pre-germ era*: characterized by a rudimentary knowledge of anatomy and physiology, of what 'goes on' inside the body and what causes disease. This lasted until the 1850s

- *Germ era*: characterized by the emergence of germ theory (Lister and Pasteur) and the concomitant rise of scientific medicine and the biomedical model

- *Post-germ era*: the realization that there are profound limitations in concentrating the whole of disease in the area of the germ being the causative agent. Germ theory does little to explain psychiatric illness, chronic illness and socially engineered diseases (e.g. exposure to toxic industrial chemicals)

Biomedical model

The biomedical model is reductionist in form, seeking explanations of dysfunction in invariant biological structures and processes. It privileges such explanations at the expense of social, cultural and biographical (life history) explanations. In its clinical mode, this dominant model of medical reasoning implies (Atkinson 1988):

- that diseases exist as distinct entities
- that those entities are revealed through the inspection of 'signs' and 'symptoms'
- that the individual patient is a more or less passive site of disease manifestation
- that diseases are to be understood as categorical departures or deviations from 'normality'.

Criticisms of the biomedical model

Tied closely to this model is the belief that medical scientific knowledge is objective. It is interesting to note the recent emphasis on evidence-based practice, which suggests that, for many medical and surgical interventions, there is no conclusive supporting evidence. In addition, Helman (1995) argues that the way in which diseases are perceived is not homogeneous and that different specialisms within medicine will view 'disease' from a number of, often very different, perspectives. Disability activists in particular have been critical of the medical model (see Chapter 15), and a number of other challenges can be identified (Gabe et al 1994):

- the managerial challenge to medical dominance
- the challenge of a more sophisticated nursing profession
- the increased rate of litigation
- the increase in media investigation
- the increase in alternative therapies
- the rise in the number of self-help groups
- more importance being attached to 'lay beliefs'
- the influence of feminist movements in the health field.

In addition to the challenges to medicine's status and claim to objectivity, there has also been doubt cast on its usefulness. McKeown (1976) demonstrated that the fall in the incidence of infectious diseases at the end of the nineteenth century was due more to higher standards of living, hygiene and nutrition than to any immunization programmes that had been introduced, and the McKinlays (1977) and Kass (1971) showed, similarly, that major declines in mortality preceded the particular treatments of modern medicine. However, a critique of these arguments has been made by Szreter (1988), who argues that McKeown has overemphasized airborne disease, respiratory tuberculosis and the decline in smallpox owing to vaccination. On the contrary, says Szreter, one group of airborne diseases – bronchitis, pneumonia and influenza – actually increased.

Other sociological criticisms of the biomedical model have come from Ivan Illich and from Marxists such as Navarro.

Illich and Navarro

Illich (1975) sees medicine as essentially a negative and damaging influence because of its iatrogenic effects. By iatrogenesis, Illich means that the medical system can produce side-effects that are detrimental to the individual; for example, too many antibiotics can have highly negative effects on the individual's ability to provide an immunity against certain 'germs'. He also identifies different types of iatrogenesis (Box 10.2).

Navarro, on the other hand, is less critical of medicine itself. His emphasis, from a Marxist perspective, is on the need to change the patterns of control over the economic and political system. Both Navarro (1976) and Waitzkin (1983) tie the evils of disease, medicine and illness firmly

---

Box 10.2   Iatrogenesis (Illich 1975)

- *Clinical iatrogenesis*: physical damage caused by the physician (side-effects of operations and medication)
- *Social iatrogenesis*: the belief that medicine is the answer to everything ('a pill for every ill')
- *Structural iatrogenesis*: the patient's loss of autonomy (the dominance of health agencies)

together with the evils of capitalism. Any improvements in the health system necessitate fundamental changes in the structure of society. The same is true of health in developing countries, where it is plain to see that economic development is closely tied to an improvement in morbidity and mortality statistics.

Feminism and medicine

The sexuality of women has traditionally been viewed by medicine as threatening and disruptive, the female body often being portrayed as an inferior version of the male body. The history of gynaecology is seen by feminists as a history of women's subservience wrapped in the guise of scientific objectivity. Thus pregnancy, menstruation, the menopause and hysteria have all been used historically (and some would claim are still being used) to instil a patriarchal ideology and keep women in a subservient position (Turner 1987).

More recent challenges to biomedicine have come from a postmodernist perspective.

The rise of postmodernism

Social theorists have, over the past 20 years, begun to talk of the end of modernity and the rise of postmodernism. By this, they mean that the ideas that people took for granted in the nineteenth and first half of the twentieth century, such as a universal 'truth', the 'objectivity' of rational science, the idea of 'progress' and so on, are no longer valid. Nettleton (1995, p. 34) sums it up thus:

postmodernism represents a break with modernism, denying any single truth or reality and emphasising the coexistence of multiple realities ... there is a loss of faith in a single, coherent, unified, linear and progressive account of the past. Instead of a legitimate 'history' there are many histories which, in turn, tend to focus less on significant events and more on the mundane aspects of everyday life.

The consequence of this approach to a sociology of health and illness is that 'expert' knowledge is no more valid than 'lay' knowledge, and the biomedical model no more valid than 'folk' models for explaining health and disease.

Activity 10.2

What are the implications of a plurality of knowledge systems and explanations for practising therapists?

Lay perspectives on health and illness

The World Health Organisation (WHO) gives a very broad definition of health, describing it as a positive state of physical, psychological and social well-being (Taylor & Field 1993). Sociologists believe, as we have seen, that illness is socially constructed, by which they mean that we construct health and illness through, and out of, our personal experiences. They highlight that the way in which we think of health is subject to variation. Thus Blaxter & Paterson (1982) found that 'health' can be defined in a number of ways, including the absence of illness (negative definition), being physically fit and being able to do certain things (functional definition). Variations in the definition of health are also related to social status, and studies in the UK, such as those of Calnan (1987) and Williams (1990), have demonstrated the wide range of ideas upon which people draw to 'make sense' of their illnesses.

Activity 10.3

What does being healthy mean to you? Do you think that you are healthy?

Having dealt briefly with problems surrounding 'health', we find similar difficulties if we turn to 'illness'. One of the first distinctions we need to make is between illness and disease. The concept of disease is associated with the biomedical model. We find that it is claimed to be arrived at by 'objective' and 'scientific' procedures, resulting in diagnosis. Illness, on the other hand, is more of a lay term and subject to people's different interpretations and reactions. Conflict can arise in health settings when the doctor uses the 'language of disease' and the patient the 'language of illness'. Health workers often find themselves in the role of 'mediator' or 'translator' between the two (Taylor & Field 1993).

The illness iceberg

This difference between illness and disease is also reflected in the way in which people seek help. The concept of the 'illness iceberg' describes a phenomenon whereby most people who perceive symptoms are not seen by medical practitioners. A study carried out in South London (Wadsworth et al 1971) found that 91% of subjects reported some form of symptom. Of these, just over half were doing something about their symptoms other than seeing health professionals, and just over a quarter were doing nothing at all. Rather than consult doctors, people will use folk remedies (e.g. whisky, lemon and honey for a cold) or over-the-counter medication (e.g. paracetamol). The concept of the illness iceberg suggests that there is a lot of 'disease' in the community that goes undiagnosed.

Activity 10.4

What did you do last time you felt 'ill'? If you went to see a doctor, at what point did you decide to do so?

Consultation triggers

Activity 10.4 highlights an important issue: the fact that seeking medical help is not just dependent on pain and discomfort. Zola (1973) identified a number of triggers to consultation, which included:

- previous experience of the condition
- interference with work
- interference with social/leisure activities.

Another important issue identified by Zola and others was the role played by others, such as relatives and friends, in encouraging and legitimating medical consultation ('You should get that seen to!').

Of course, the above factors are not the only ones implicated in the seeking of medical help or the frequency with which it is sought. Age, sex, class and ethnic group can all be influential. Worsley (1987) highlights research showing that women consult more than men, working-class men are more likely to consult than middle-class men, and middle-class women are more likely to seek immunization and health check-ups for their children. Worsley cautions that this research needs to be read critically. For example, feminists have highlighted the increasing involvement and control by medicine over women's bodies, leading to greater pressure to consult. Working-class men may consult more because they need to get absences certified, whereas middle-class men are subject to less control and scrutiny in the workplace. We also need to remember that the general living conditions of the working classes – more dangerous manual jobs and poorer housing – are more likely to produce ill-health.

So far we have looked at factors leading to medical consultations; it is now time to turn our attention to what happens when doctors (and other health professionals) meet their patients.

THE MEDICAL ENCOUNTER

It is possible to identify a number of different approaches to the medical encounter. First, there is the functionalist perspective. In contrast to this, there is an approach focusing on the power differential between doctor and patient, and there are also more interactionist perspectives that examine medical encounters as arenas of negotiation.

Functionalist approach

Here, the relationship between patient and professional is not seen in terms of conflict, as a power struggle between lay people and professionals, but as a harmonious one. Parsons' notion of the sick role typifies this perspective. You will remember from Chapter 5 that the sick role confers on patients certain rights and responsibilities. Doctors are also subject to certain duties and 'rights', for example that they will have specialized knowledge and that they will be deferred to. Another variation of the functionalist approach comes from Szasz & Hollender (1956, cited in Morgan et al 1985). They identify three types of doctor–patient relationship, which vary with the nature of the problem encountered. An 'active–passive' relationship exists in situations in which the patient is unable to respond (e.g. coma). Here the doctor does things to the patient. The 'guidance–cooperation' relationship is typical of acute illnesses, the doctor telling the patient what to do and the patient being expected to comply. Finally, a 'mutual participation' relationship exists, in which the doctor still provides the expert help but also helps patients to help themselves. Szasz & Hollender believed this relationship to be typical of chronic illness.

A conflict perspective

Friedson (1970) has been particularly critical of the functionalist perspective on the doctor–patient relationship. He argues that theorists such as Parsons and Szasz & Hollender describe the relationship as doctors would *like* it to be. In actual fact, there is a tension in the relationship between the doctor, who approaches the patient in terms of a clinical case to be diagnosed and treated, and the patient, who comes with a cultural background and demands of managing a daily life. Friedson acknowledges that, in some circumstances, it may actually be the patient who guides the doctor.

Activity 10.5

What is the nature of your relationship with your doctor? Is it one of equality or medical dominance?

It could, of course, be argued that Friedson's work is now rather dated and that attempts have been made to educate doctors (and other professionals) more rigorously with respect to interpersonal and communication skills. However, a recent British report (Baker et al 1997) has highlighted the fact that disabled people do not feel that professionals fully recognize that they are not just 'patients'. The message coming across from disabled people was that they are handicapped by social attitudes and not sufficiently involved in the planning of their care. This adds weight to the criticism that the existence of a participative relationship between doctor and patient is more of an ideal than a reality.

Power relations in medical encounters

It seems, then, that patients often leave the medical encounter with their perceived needs, particularly for information, unmet. Even when highly motivated, doctors tend to underestimate patients' desire for information and to overestimate their own communicative skills. Communication barriers seem greatest when professionals and clients of different class background, sex or race try to interact (Waitzkin 1983, p. 143).

Amir (1980), in a discussion of the social organization of a visit to the doctor, sees the doctor–patient interaction as only one aspect of the situation. For example, there are special settings (examination room, waiting room and doctor's room), complying with procedures (making an appointment) and dealing with a number of people (receptionist and nurse). These are all part of the experience and can add to the disempowering of the patient.

Power in the relationship is sustained in a number of ways. The functionalists would say that the patient must acquiesce to what the physician tells him to do. He becomes a 'case', the 'patient', passive and eager to comply with the medical regimen. Doctors not only exercise power, but also do so in an increasing number of areas of life. Medicalization refers to the process whereby power and control are applied by the medical profession to areas not essentially or intrinsically medical, such as childbirth, obesity and alcohol use, in which technical or biomedical 'solutions' are foisted on what are regarded often as 'normal' manifestations of everyday life and are attempts at increased social regulation.

There is, however, another perspective, which views the medical encounter as one of neither consensus nor dominance. Some very enlightening work has been undertaken by sociologists working within a symbolic interactionist tradition. This work sees the medical encounter as one of negotiation.

An interactionist perspective

This approach is highlighted in the literature on chronic illness, particularly the management of chronic pain. Baszanger (1989) uses the term 'work' to describe the efforts of participants in medical situations:

> The medical work of managing chronic illness brings together physicians and patients over an extended period. In this sense there is not a relationship but a *succession, over time, of interactions* with a common purpose – managing the illness – which although it may initially set the principal parties at odds, does generally bring them together.

The work of the patient is particularly difficult, especially in hospital, in the early stages of chronic illness. Here, medical staff tend to be focused on diagnosing and treating the disease. Part of the problem the patient faces is in communicating her level of pain because pain is a perception not amenable to any diagnostic test. Indeed, in some circumstances, there may not even be any accompanying observable pathology. The patient is faced with the task of convincing medical staff of the legitimacy of the pain. If the patient adopts the wrong tactic, for example being very vociferous, she runs the risk of being labelled a demanding or difficult patient. If she underplays the pain, professionals may underestimate its severity. Fagerhaugh & Strauss (1977) found that both nurses and physiotherapists underestimated the severity of low back pain in certain patients. The reason why staff may ignore expressions of pain is that it does not fit with what they consider normal. The ideas that staff carry with them of what is an expected level of pain in a certain condition has been called the 'pain trajectory'.

So far, we have been talking mainly about physical conditions. An important concept that grew out of Goffman's work on psychiatric services is the patient career.

THE PATIENT CAREER

Through his work on psychiatric institutions, Goffman (1961) developed the notion of the moral career of the 'mental' patient. He described how patients progress through a process of recognition of symptoms, diagnosis, treatment and outcome of treatment. Through this process, the person undergoes a change in status and identity. Thus a person may start his 'career' as a bank clerk and end it as a mental patient or ex-mental patient. Along the way, he learns how to behave as a patient (complying with doctors' requests, etc.), and others begin to respond to him as a patient rather than to his previous identity. Although this concept was initially developed in relation to mental illness, the same process can be seen in physical settings, both acute and chronic (Bond & Bond 1994). These notions of becoming a patient and of change in identity are also evident in the work of writers who have talked of biographical disruption.

Biographical disruption

Most of us have a sense of who we are and, to a greater or lesser extent, where our lives are going; that is to say, we have some consciousness of our history and our future – our biography. The onset of chronic illness can present a form of disruption to that biography. Very often, it means a revision of future plans and events in the past. Thus one does not just have a chronic illness; it has particular meaning and significance. Bury (1988) distinguishes between 'meaning as consequence', which is the practical problems that a condition throws up, and 'meaning as significance', which is more to do with the way in which people view the condition. In most Western cultures, chronic illness is still viewed as something that is to be pitied, the individual being protected from the challenges of everyday life. If people attempt to continue with their normal life, they run the risk of having their claim to being ill disbelieved. This is particularly true for people with chronic pain or chronic fatigue syndrome, in which there may be no visible impairment.

Kotarba (1983) has also focused on the process of becoming a person with chronic pain. He identified three stages in the process (Box 10.3).

The work of Bury and Kotarba belongs to a school of thought that adopts a phenomenological perspective on the body. This is particularly to be seen in patients' narratives, i.e. the way in which they tell others about their chronic illness (Kleinman 1988). Here, illness is viewed as being particularly separated from disease (the 'objective', 'scientific' construct) and is instead

---

Box 10.3 Becoming a chronic pain sufferer

1. *Onset*: The person and medical staff attempt to treat and diagnose the pain, which is accepted as real
2. *Emergence of doubt*: Initial investigations and treatment having proved unsuccessful, the patient moves into a cycle of ever more specialist consultations and investigations
3. *Chronic pain experience*: Patients begin to seek other, lay, explanations for their condition. They enter a chronic pain subculture

---

peculiarly human and reflective. By this, we mean that animals have diseases but that they do not think about their meaning or significance; they do not 'have illnesses'. The incapacity of the body makes us reflect on the experience of illness. This differs from the majority of times when we take for granted the body's capabilities. The body is therefore not a passive entity but an interactive and reflective one.

LESSONS FOR OCCUPATIONAL THERAPY

The material covered in this chapter highlights three particular issues of importance to therapists. The first relates to consultation triggers, the second to 'encounters' with clients and the third to the impact of chronic illness on self-identity and the implications of this for therapeutic intervention. A case study relating to a person with chronic pain will be used as an illustration (Case study 10.1).

Chronic pain has been chosen because it is a feature of many conditions that occupational therapists encounter in their daily practice. At the same time, it is one that is poorly understood by health and social care professionals. This is beginning to change, as shown by the increasing number of books by occupational therapists on the subject (O'Hara, 1996, Strong 1996). These books should be consulted to discover more about the specific therapeutic intervention relevant to the case study as we will only deal with the sociological aspects here.

Case study 10.1 A person with chronic pain

Mary is a 34-year-old night-club security officer. She has been off work for the past 6 months because of low back pain, beginning when she was involved in a scuffle after refusing someone admission. She initially took 2 weeks rest and then returned to work. The pain persisted, and when she returned to work, she found it difficult to fulfil her duties, although she was reluctant to admit it, and was eventually assigned an administrative job. She put up with the pain for a few months but eventually went back to the doctor when she found it increasingly difficult to play with her 3-year-old child or make love with her husband. Her relationship with her husband has begun to suffer, and he feels that she is using her pain as an excuse to reject him. Despite seeing a physiotherapist and self-referral to a reflexologist, the pain worsened and Mary has been signed off work. Further tests have not shown anything significant, and Mary's doctor thinks that the pain may be 'psychological' and linked to the original circumstances of her injury. Mary is unwilling to see a psychiatrist but accepts being referred to a pain management programme. However, there is a 6-month waiting period, and in the meantime, she has been referred to an occupational therapist for advice on making daily living tasks easier.

CONSULTATION TRIGGERS

Mary, in Case study 10.1, represents a good example of the type of situation described above by Zola, i.e. that it is not necessarily pain or discomfort that acts as a trigger for help seeking but interference with valued activities. This has important implications, particularly in the case of chronic pain sufferers. The longer that people attempt to struggle on, the greater the danger of longlasting neurological changes taking place, which may make the pain more intractable. It is increasingly recognized that early intervention in chronic pain is important (Jensen & Rasmussen 1994).

Another factor that may have led Mary to delay consultation is her membership of a particular occupational subculture.

OCCUPATIONAL SUBCULTURE

Kotarba (1983) illustrated the importance of occupational subculture in relation to athletes and manual workers. In both instances, he highlighted how pain is a common aspect of their daily working life and how admission of it can be a threat to employment and self-image. For Mary, as a woman in a traditionally male occupation, she may have been under particular pressure to show that she could 'take the knocks' as well as (if not better than) her male colleagues. Kotarba (1983, p. 134) states, 'The pain afflicted person may decide to conceal the experience of pain from potentially critical audiences if the social and emotional costs resulting from disclosure outweigh the perceived benefits.'

Activity 10.6

Make a list of occupations in which reporting pain could pose the dilemmas highlighted by Kotarba.

ENCOUNTERS WITH THERAPISTS

Unless therapists have a good understanding of the neurological mechanisms involved in pain, they may be in danger of responding inappropriately. In Mary's case this would be:

- believing the pain to be psychogenic
- believing that the best thing to do would be to reduce the number of activities required of her and introducing unnecessary aids and adaptations.

A study of women with chronic pain by Howell (1994) illustrated the devastating effect of the failure of health-care professionals to accept a person's pain as real. This is a particular danger in conditions such as low back pain, in which it may be difficult to identify pathological changes (tissue damage, etc.). Such negative responses led to women becoming increasingly isolated and focused on their pain.

In contrast to the above negative approaches, the women in Howell's study found it most helpful when professionals and others accepted the bodily reality of their pain and they were helped to lead a fulfilling life despite their pain or, as Howell conceptualized it, 'fulfilling my life with pain'. An important role for the therapist could be to educate Mary and her husband or empower them with information about the possible factors involved in her chronic pain and why tests may not be able to find physical damage. Rather than reducing Mary's activity levels, the therapist would suggest pacing and goal-setting and relaxation techniques, and utilize a knowledge of ergonomics and biomechanics to enable a return to valued activities.

This type of approach highlights the notion of 'medical work' discussed earlier in this chapter. The concept of a negotiated relationship is one that fits very comfortably with the philosophy of occupational therapy. However, in reality, the therapist's relationship with Mary may not take this form because of the nature of the agency employing the therapist. Thus the focus of the agency may be on assessment and the provision of aids and adaptations rather than on more long-term therapeutic intervention. In this situation, there may be a tension between what Mary wants (to get back to doing what she likes) and what the therapist is offering (equipment or personal support, e.g. home help).

Activity 10.7

Can you think of any non-biomedical explanations of illness or health remedies that are common in your own cultural group?

Have you come across any situations in which what the therapist had to offer was not what the client wanted? How was this situation resolved? Was any compromise reached?

So far we have mainly been dealing with what Bury (1988) called 'meaning as consequence', i.e. the practical problems caused by chronic pain. In order to claim to be practising holistically, we also need to consider 'meaning as significance'. In helping Mary to rebuild her life, the therapist is engaged in helping to construct a new biography, that is to say, helping Mary to create a positive self-identity rather than slide into a negative one.

SELF-IDENTITY

Mary would appear to be following the process of becoming a chronic pain sufferer, as identified by Kotarba and outlined above. If intervention takes place at stage 2, therapy will clearly be easier than in stage 3.

For many people with chronic pain, it is not possible to remove the pain, although some reduction may be possible. Indeed, one of the problems faced by pain management programmes is that of working with people who are locked into searching for a 'cure'. This is reflected in the findings of Howell (1994, p. 108), who noted that some women in her study 'devoted themselves to finding "the cure" and trying "everything possible" to rid themselves of having pain that destroyed their ways of relating to themselves as people and with others'. In contrast, the women who coped best with their pain were those who felt that they had a fulfilling and healthy life *despite* their pain. This again emphasizes the different ways in which people conceptualize being healthy, as discussed earlier in this chapter, and the importance of enabling meaningful occupations.

CONCLUSION

This chapter has covered only a few aspects of a major area of sociology. We have looked at the different models of health and illness and how the way in which people think about these concepts can be at odds with medical perspectives. We have highlighted the different ways of looking at the relationship between health-care professionals and their clients, i.e. as one of consensus, conflict or negotiation. Of particular interest to occupational therapists is the way in which sociological studies can illuminate the process that leads people to seek help. Awareness of this is important in developing early intervention strategies.

In particular, we have focused on the way in which the sociology of chronic illness can help us to analyse the situation of people with chronic pain. Phenomenological approaches to 'the body' can help us to avoid the mind/body split identified by Bendelow & Williams (1995). Such an approach can highlight the interaction between mind, body and the individual's place in society. The literature can sensitize us to issues that may affect both the relationship between therapist and client and the focus of intervention. This field of sociology supports therapeutic practice that is biopsychosocial in nature.

REFERENCES

Amir D 1980 The social organisation of a visit to the doctor. In: Roth J (ed.) Research in the Sociology of Health. Aijai Press, Greenwich, CT

Atkinson P 1988 Discourse descriptions and diagnoses reproducing normal medicine. In Lock M, Gordon D (eds) Biomedicine examined. Kluwer Academic, London.

Baker M, Fardell J, Jones B 1997 Disability and rehabilitation: survey of education needs of health and social service professionals. Disability and Rehabilitation Open Learning Project, London

Baszanger I 1989 Pain: its experience and treatments. Social Science and Medicine 29(3): 425–434

Bendelow G A, Williams S J 1995 Transcending the dualisms: towards a sociology of pain. Sociology of Health and Illness 17(2): 139–165

Blaxter M, Paterson E 1982 Mothers and daughters: a three generational study of attitudes and behaviour. Heineman, London.

Bond J, Bond S 1994 Sociology and health care: an introduction for nurses and other health care professionals, 2nd edn. Churchill Livingstone, Edinburgh

Bury M 1988 Meanings at risk. In: Anderson R, Bury M (eds) Living with chronic illness: the experience of patients and their families. Hyman Unwin, London.

Calnan M 1987 Health and illness: the lay perspective. Tavistock, London.

Fagerhaugh S Y, Strauss A 1977 Politics of pain management: staff patient interaction. Addison-Wesley, Menlo Park, CA

Freund P, McGuire M 1995 Health, illness and the social body. Prentice Hall, New Jersey

Friedson E 1970 The profession of medicine. Dodd Mead, New York

Gabe J, Kelleher, D, Williams G (eds) 1994 Challenging medicine. Routledge, London

Goffman E 1961 Asylum: essays on the social situation of mental patients and other inmates. Anchor Books, New York

Helman C G 1995 Culture health and illness, 3rd edn. Butterworth, London.

Howell S L 1994 A theoretical model for caring for women with chronic nonmalignant pain. Qualitative Health Research 4(1): 94–122

Illich I 1975 Medical nemesis: the expropriation of health. Calder & Boyers, London

Jensen T S, Rasmussen P 1994 Phantom pain and related phenomena after amputation. In: Wall P D, Melzack R (eds) Textbook of pain. Churchill Livingstone, London.

Kass E 1971 Infectious diseases and social change. Journal of Infectious Diseases 123: 110–114

Kleinman A 1988 The illness narratives: suffering, healing and the human condition. Basic Books, New York

Kotarba J 1983 Chronic pain: its social dimensions. Sage, Thousand Oaks, California

Lupton D 1994 Medicine as culture: illness, disease and the body in Western societies. Sage, London

McKeown T 1976 The role of medicine: dream, mirage or nemesis? Nuffield Provincial Hospitals Trust, London

McKinlay J, McKinlay S 1977 The questionable contribution of medical measures to the decline of mortality in the United States in the twentieth century. Health and Society 53: 1

Morgan M, Calnan M, Manning N 1985 Sociological approaches to health and medicine. Croom Helm, London

Navarro V 1976 Medicine under capitalism. Croom Helm, London

Nettleton S 1995 The sociology of health and illness. Polity Press, London

O'Hara P 1996 Pain management for health professionals. Chapman & Hall, London

Strong J 1996 Chronic pain: the occupational therapist's perspective. Churchill Livingstone, London

Szasz T, Hollender M H 1956 A contribution to the philosophy of medicine. AMA Archives of Internal Medicine XCVII: 585–592

Szreter S 1988 The importance of social intervention in Britain's mortality decline c1850–1914: a reinterpretation of the role of public health. In: Davey B, Gray A, Seale C (eds) Health and disease: a reader. Open University Press, Buckingham 1994

Taylor S, Field D 1993 Sociology of health and health care: an introduction for nurses. Blackwell Scientific, London

Turner B 1987 Medical power and social knowledge. Sage, London

Wadsworth M, Butterfield W, Blaney R 1971 Health and sickness: the choice of treatment. Tavistock, London

Waitzkin H 1983 The second sickness. Free Press, New York

Williams R 1990 The Protestant legacy: attitudes towards death and illness among older Aberdonians. Oxford University Press, Oxford

Worsley P 1987 The new introducing sociology. Penguin, Harmondsworth

Zola I K 1973 Pathways to the doctor from person to patient. Social Science and Medicine 2: 677–689

11

Organizations

Carol Lennie   Linda B. M. Renton

THE IMPORTANCE OF ORGANIZATIONS

Organizations are part of everyday life. It is difficult to think of activities that are not to some extent influenced by an organization, from our taste in food to our work. In this chapter, we will examine the impact of organizations and how they work in terms of achieving goals and controlling their members, and we will focus on the individual within the organization. The second part of this chapter looks at the implications for therapists of working within organizations, be they statutory or voluntary, concerned with health or social care. A discussion of selected issues will enable you to think about how working in an organization affects you as a therapist. However, we first need to attempt to define what we mean by the term 'organization'.

DEFINING ORGANIZATIONS

Owing to the complexities of organizations, there are numerous approaches to defining them. The five approaches listed below are by no means the only approaches but will give a flavour of the range of views. It is important to note that the definition used will have a direct effect on our focus when studying organizations.

Goal achievement

One way of thinking about organizations is to see them as an attempt to realize clearly defined goals. A number of theorists have taken this approach. For example, Etzioni defined organizations as 'planned units, deliberately structured for the purpose of attaining specific goals' (Etzioni 1964, p. 4). Sofer (1972) saw organizations as being made up of 'associations of people' grouped together around specific goals. He argued that this meant that individuals could achieve objectives that they could not achieve on their own. However, this emphasis on 'specific goals' as a defining criterion may be problematic given that goals may change over a period of time.

Composition

An alternative to looking at organizations as goal-directed units is to see them as being composed of identifiable members. Caplow (1964, p. 1), following this approach, defined an organization as 'a social system that has an unequivocal collective identity, an exact roster of members, a programme of activity and procedures'. However, the notion of 'an exact roster of members' being characteristic of an organization may be questioned. For example, are churches organizations given that they do not keep exact rosters of members?

Goals and functions

Classifying organizations according to their goals and functions is typical of a functionalist approach. Parsons (1960), using these criteria, placed organizations into four main categories:

- economic production
- political goals
- pattern maintenance (e.g. education)
- integration (e.g. police).

The main problem with this type of approach is that organizations do not necessarily fall into only one category, and there may be disagreements over which category they do fit into.

Organizations as systems

This approach views an organization as being made up of interlocking and interacting parts. There are a number of different types of system within an organization, such as information systems, formal social systems and informal social systems. This approach highlights two important areas within organizational studies: first, the methods used to control or organize members of an organization, and second, the fact that organizations exist as part of the wider systems of community, national and international political and economic systems, all of which may affect them. These issues are considered below.

Organizational typologies

Instead of aiming at a general definition, some authors have found it more effective to examine a range of organizations and create a list of the properties that they hold. Merton (1952), for example, listed 26 shared properties of organizations. It is also possible to use typologies to identify differences between organizations in terms of structure, systems of control, communication, etc.

However, no matter what approach to definition we take, it is vital to remember that organizations are made up of people. There is a general tendency to talk about organizations as if they are an actual entity that speaks and acts. This masks the reality that it is individuals within those organizations who make the decisions, and ignoring this allows individuals to avoid responsibility for their actions.

Organizations themselves both affect and are affected by individual members. Informal organization exists within formal organizations where individuals develop their own way of doing things and groups form their own codes of conduct, which may be different from those officially given.

ORGANIZATIONAL IMPACTS

We have already suggested that it is the case that organizations affect individuals and wider society, and it is this aspect that we will examine next. We will look at the effect on the individual, the family, the community and the social structure.

Individual

Work organizations tend to shape us more than do most groups to which we belong. This is partly because their influence is highly specific, in that we know how we are expected to behave. Work organizations have systematic training procedures to ensure that members fit into their roles. Alongside training procedures, there are rules and obligations as well as informal pressures. This combination of factors can have an effect on our personal values.

Activity 11.1

Have your studies and training altered any of your prior views towards clients and/or other professional groups alongside whom you work?

According to Hall (1972), the most important outcome of organizations for individuals is where they are placed within the social stratification system. In other words, the type of job we hold within an organization gives us our socioeconomic status, which in turn has a direct effect on our own and our family's life chances. Organizations also reflect the divisions in society, so it is not surprising that women and ethnic minority groups find themselves subject to vertical and horizontal segregation in work organizations.

Family

Eldridge & Crombie (1974) noted that work organizations affect family relationships and family structure. For example, work organizations determine where employees will live, which in turn affects how much contact can be maintained with the family of origin (i.e. the family that the person was born into). The number of hours worked and when these hours are to be worked will influence the time that individuals have to spend with their family. In recent years, many commentators have expressed concern over the impact that long hours of work demanded by organizations will have on families.

Community

Organizations have a direct impact on the local communities in which they are located. These organizations may dominate an area in terms of their influence on the local economy, housing and job markets. Having a high-status organization in the community can also alter the status of the community itself: consider the effect of having a large government department or the head office of a multinational conglomerate situated in a particular locality.

Social structure

If organizations have important outcomes for individuals and communities, it is obvious that they also have important outcomes for the wider society in which they are embedded. Large industrial organizations are of crucial importance in Western economies. They play an enormous part in economic planning within modern societies. As J. K. Galbraith (1972) has pointed out, where massive commitments are made, organizations cannot afford to leave their markets to chance. In other words, large industrial organizations wield political as well as economic power. The fact that organizations enable a relatively few people to have massive economic and political power has been of concern to many sociologists. Blau & Scott (1963), writing in the 1960s, warned that large organizations were a threat to democracies. Other theorists, such as Salaman (1979), have focused on the perpetuation of class differences through organizational structures.

It is not just industrial organizations that have political power; arguably, organizations such as hospitals, schools and social work departments are also important. Broadly speaking, these organizations can be seen as maintaining and legitimating existing patterns of inequality and exploitation. They reflect the values of the ruling

---

Activity 11.2

Have changes in social policy and legislation affected the service that you can give or the nature of health and social care organizations you come across?

---

class, for example in their support of the nuclear family, and primarily protect their interests. It could be argued that their role is to maintain the *status quo* by supplying a service apparently available equally to all. They provide the sticking plaster for a society that would otherwise fall apart, but they do not deal with the origins of social problems.

BUREAUCRACY

As organizations become larger and more complex, they require a structure that can direct, coordinate and control the activities of the many people engaged in the diversity of different tasks. According to Max Weber, bureaucratic organizations are ordered into a hierarchy that takes the shape of a pyramid-type structure based on a division of function and authority. Weber believed that bureaucracies were the most efficient organizational structure. He argued that:

The decisive reason for the advance of bureaucratic organisation has always been its purely technical superiority over any other form of organisation. The fully developed bureaucratic mechanism compares with other organisations exactly, as does the machine with the non mechanical modes of production. (cited in Gerth & Mills 1948, p. 214)

Weber held that bureaucracy was more rational in terms of control being exercised on the basis of knowledge, expertise and technical competence. This would in turn lead to a stable and calculable administration, which was essential for any kind of large organization. Thus this organizational type was likely to continue to expand.

Yet in popular discourse, bureaucracy is synonymous with inefficiency rather than rationality and efficiency. Thus government ministers seeking to improve their popularity will promise to cut back on 'red tape'. To understand this discrepancy, we need to examine bureaucracy further.

Bureaucracy as an ideal type

To emphasize the differences between bureaucracies and other types of organization, Weber created an 'ideal type', which demonstrated that bureaucracy was the most effective structure

---

Box 11.1   Weber's 'ideal-type' organization

1. *Specialization*: Workers are familiar with and responsible for only one area of work. They have a clearly defined sphere of competence

2. *Hierarchy*: In organizations, this consists of positions or offices rather than people. Authority rests in the office, not in the person who occupies it. Each person is responsible to the person directly above in the chain of command and responsible for the actions of those below. In addition, the authority of these individual offices is clearly defined and limited

3. *Rules*: Activities and relationships in a bureaucracy are governed by explicit rules

4. *Impersonality*: Personal emotions get in the way of efficiency, and officials should conduct their office *sine ira et studio* – without hatred or passion – and hence without affection or enthusiasm

5. *Appointed officials*: The basis of appointments is technical competence; they get the post through merit

6. *Full-time officials*: The post should be the sole or main occupation of the holder

7. *Career officials*: There is a system of promotion according to seniority, merit or both. This is essential to motivate individuals and create an *esprit de corps*

8. *Private/public split*: Members of a bureaucracy cannot own any of its resources

---

to meet administrative objectives. It should be noted that an 'ideal type' is not a description of a real organization or even what it should be but is a theoretical tool allowing sociologists to abstract features found in all large-scale organizations. Weber's ideal type included the features found in Box 11.1.

If all the features of Weber's ideal type were present, this would in theory lead to a competent staff who gained their position through merit. Decisions would be taken on the basis of laid-down criteria ensuring equitable treatment for all. Complex organizations could be made orderly and predictable through rules being followed.

Problems with bureaucracy

Despite this, Weber recognized that bureaucracies had failings. He talked of the 'paradox of consequences' whereby highly rational procedures could divert from the original values that had inspired them. His greatest concern, however, was the effect that bureaucracies had on those working in them. He noted:

each man becomes a little cog in the machine and aware of this, his one preoccupation is whether he can become a bigger cog ... it is horrible to think that the world could one day be filled with these little cogs, little men clinging to little jobs, and striving towards bigger ones ... the passion for bureaucracy is enough to drive one to despair. (cited in Mayer 1956, p. 127)

Bureaucracy and organizational efficiency

Weber was not the only theorist to raise concerns over both the impact of bureaucracy on individuals and the effect that bureaucratic procedures have on original organizational goals. Merton (1952) was especially interested in the latter concern and, in his study 'The nature and sources of pathological bureaucratic behaviour', examined the inbuilt failings that are found in such organizational structures. He believed that bureaucracies, as defined by Weber's ideal type, would lead to red tape and rigidity, leaving organizations incapable of coping with change. He was aware that following bureaucratic procedures would lead to reliability and the predictability of organizational members, thus making them easier for management to control. However, this was also likely to lead to inflexibility and the displacement of organizational goals. Merton described the process of 'trained incapacity', in which organizational members are trained to strictly follow and adhere to rules, and how when bureaucracies were faced with problems resulting from following rules, they created further rules to deal with this. He referred to this as a 'bureaucratic vicious circle'. The problem that Merton clearly identified was that if organizational members are rewarded for following rules, they are likely to become devoted to procedures, turning them into rituals rather than questioning the consequences of following these procedures in all cases.

Satirists have also very effectively questioned the rationality and efficiency of Weber's ideal type. C. Northcote Parkinson (1958) created 'Parkinson's Law', which states that 'Work ex-

pands to fill the time available for its completion.' Thus, far from being efficient, bureaucracies create meaningless tasks simply to look busy! Similarly, Laurence Peter and Raymond Hull (1969) questioned whether bureaucracies did make optimum use of talent and expertise. They created the 'Peter Principle', which states that 'In a hierarchy, every employee tends to rise to his own level of incompetence.' In other words, people are promoted until they reach the point at which the post exceeds their ability.

Informal structures within bureaucracies

Several studies of actual bureaucratic organizations imply that Merton overstated his case, as they found informal networks in which organizational members did bend the rules. In addition, this behaviour was not necessarily to the detriment of the organization and might indeed have promoted the overall goals of the organization.

Blau's (1956) famous study of the Federal Law Enforcement Agency demonstrated how an informal system aided the overall efficiency of the organization. Under official rules, agents were not allowed to discuss cases with colleagues and were required to discuss them only with a supervisor. To have followed this rigidly would have meant agents working in isolation and without support, as they were unlikely to jeopardize future promotion by constantly asking for help. Instead, agents did discuss cases with colleagues. This had the effect of pooling information and expertise, which led to greater efficiency.

In a similar vein, Lipsky (1980) studied social workers and developed the concept of 'street-level bureaucracy'. This refers to the way in which practitioners have to work with legislation and policy handed down from above. Workers in direct contact with clients are very often forced to reinterpret or even ignore some policies in order to deal with problems such as limited resources or huge caseloads.

Effectiveness of bureaucracies

Although Weber saw the rise of bureaucracy as inevitable, a number of theorists have questioned this view. Gouldner's (1954) study of a gypsum plant in the USA described how the factory of the plant worked under a bureaucratic structure, while the mine had a much looser informal structure. This continued despite the management's attempts to enforce a bureaucratic structure on the miners. Gouldner concluded that bureaucratic structure is more suited to routine work than to work that is unpredictable and lacking a clear routine. He also noted that workers can successfully oppose the imposition of this type of structure. Burns & Stalker (1961) came to similar conclusions on the basis of research carried out within the electronics industry in Britain.

Mechanistic and organic systems

Burns & Stalker (1961) created two ideal types of organization – the mechanistic and the organic. As you will recall from earlier discussion, organizations will not fall into these *ideal types* but will be placed somewhere in between. The mechanistic type is basically the same as Weber's ideal type. On the other hand, the organic type is not clearly defined. The hierarchy is not as rigid, communication being based on consultation rather than orders. Instead of following laid-down procedures, organizational members are encouraged to use their skills to solve problems as they arise.

Burns & Stalker argued that the mechanistic model is best suited for organizations in which there was little change, whereas organic systems are best suited to rapidly changing circumstances. They were also aware that there was a great deal of resistance to moving away from a mechanistic model, which gave some organizational members power and status, to one that might bring this into question. Bureaucracy is a structure that gives, or more accurately appears to give, management much greater control over other organizational members.

Braverman (1974) also saw bureaucracy in mechanistic terms. He argued that it became the method of management controlling the work process (and thus the workers) and led to more work being carried out for less wages. In today's language, this is referred to as efficiency!

Braverman, using Weber's imagery, argued that bureaucracy represents the implementation of mechanical principles in the organization of human activities. Bureaucracy tackles the job of administration in a way similar to that of the production line on the shop floor.

Activity 11.3

Can you think of any examples of where a bureaucratic structure, even a good one, would be inappropriate?

POWER AND CONTROL IN ORGANIZATIONS

One of the areas of greatest interest to sociologists studying organizations is the issue of power and control. Writers such as Crozier (1964) have argued that a knowledge of power relationships within organizations is essential to understanding the workings of organizations and their members. An important distinction needs to be made between the terms 'power' and 'authority' when examining organizations. Weber differentiated them as follows:

- *Power* involves force or coercion and would not normally be an important factor as an internal process in organizations except in cases such as schools, prisons and occasionally hospitals
- *Authority* involves a suspension of judgment on the part of its recipients. Instructions or orders are followed because people believe that they should be followed.

Weber's analysis is useful in that it views authority as a form of power more useful than cruder forms of power in controlling certain organizations. Since then, many writers have elaborated on different types of power used within organizations. A good example of this is a typology based on the nature of the relationship between the power-holder and the recipient that was designed by French & Raven (1959). They listed five types of power (Box 11.2).

It is obvious that different types of power are used to control organizational members; this is

Box 11.2   French and Raven's five types of power

- *Reward power* refers to where the power-holder has the ability to reward, by salary increase, promotion, etc.
- *Coercive power* is based on the recipient's perceptions of the ability of the power-holder to distribute punishments
- *Legitimate power* is similar to Weber's 'authority'
- *Referent power* is involved when a power recipient identifies with a power-holder and tries to behave like him or her
- *Expert power*

Activity 11.4

To which of the above forms of power are you subject?

true even within the same organization. It is also the case that some members of organizations are less controlled than others. For example, college lecturers have more freedom over their work than do secretarial staff. One of the most striking differences between and within organizations is the difference in the type and extent of control of the various levels of organizational members.

For employees at a low level in the organization, the basis of power is tied up to reward power in the form of remuneration. Etzioni referred to this as a 'calculative relationship'. This does not mean that this group are interested only in financial rewards, but that this is the one given prime importance. All low-level workers are likely to find themselves more closely tied up by discipline than are workers higher up in the organization. This may be because of the job itself, but it also reflects a widespread belief among management that low-level workers are less responsible and less committed to the organization.

In the case of white collar employees, research has found a level of commitment and organizational identification that is not held by low-level employees. Lockwood (1956) puts forward three possible reasons for this. First, they are more likely to have job security and a career structure. Second, their spatial situation within the organization is likely to affect their social relationships. They are unlikely to develop group solidarity

with others in the same situation as they are spread throughout the organization. This also means that they are more likely to identify with those beside whom they work, who will hold higher posts. Finally, their position within the organization gives a higher status both within and outside the organization.

Although white collar workers are more likely to identify with the organization, it does not appear to be the case that those in higher authority wholly accept this. In recent years, white collar employees have found themselves being hedged in with similar forms of control and discipline, for example clocking in and out, that are more normally associated with low-level employees.

In the case of professional and senior members, control can be argued to be a mixture of remunerative and normative methods. This group get high levels of financial remuneration, vastly superior working conditions, greater job security within a career structure and control over their own work. In addition, professional members are to some degree controlled through their commitment to professional and organizational philosophies and objectives that emphasize the importance and value of the activity in which they are involved. This means that they regulate their own work behaviour, making other methods unnecessary. Professionals, such as occupational therapists, are likely to hold convictions of the importance and necessity of their organizational activity and of their personal responsibility to undertake this with diligence and competence. This commitment is developed through their professional training, recruitment and induction into an organization.

How autonomous professionals are in reality within organizations has been questioned by Blau & Schoenherr (1971) and Salaman (1979). They both point out that professionals only have autonomy over their own particular area of expertise but have no control over the overall objectives of the organization.

Although it is clear that the control of professional and senior members of an organization is largely normative, it is also likely to be the case that this reliability and commitment would not persist long were these members not given 'appropriate levels' of financial remuneration and good working conditions. Chapter 12 explores these issues in more detail.

Activity 11.5

Are your levels of remuneration and working conditions a recognition of your professional worth? Do these affect your commitment to your post within an organization?

This emphasis on power and control appears to imply that conflict is inherent within organizations. This may be vertical conflict between members at different levels in the organization, as the ranking of non-professionals above professionals may cause insecurities and hence conflict. There may also be horizontal conflict between members at the same level, for example between different paramedical professionals over the treatment of a patient. Not all writers agree that power within organizations causes conflict. Clegg (1979) has criticized this view as it seems to assume that it is 'natural' for humans to strive for power. However, the question of power and control, with the underlying belief that this is necessary to prevent conflict within an organization, is a major focus for social scientists.

Power, bureaucracy and society

Other sociologists have been more concerned over the impact that bureaucracy has on democracy. Writers such as Michels (1921) conclude Weber to be wrong to believe that bureaucracies manage to keep authority tied to an office rather than the individual. Instead, Michels argued that bureaucracy invariably leads to the concentration of power in the hands of a few individuals who use their position in the organization to address their own ends. He termed this outcome 'The iron law of oligarchy'. Blau (1956) also took this approach, arguing that, while in a mass society democracy depends on bureaucratic institutions, these are incompatible with democracy because there would be a concentration of power in the hands of a few people, normally male.

The American political theorist Kathy Ferguson took these concerns further by picking up on the powerlessness of clients having to deal with large bureaucratic organizations and the increasing use of large organizations to control people outside the organization. She notes that 'One of the main characteristics of bureaucratic capitalism is the growing role of organisations whose sole ostensible purpose is to process, regulate, licence, certify, hide, or otherwise control individuals.' (Ferguson 1984, p. 123).

Activity 11.6

Have you experienced powerlessness when dealing with large bureaucratic organizations, for example college administration or social security? How would you address this issue in relation to patients?

This emphasis on the detrimental effects that bureaucratic types of organization have on women and men runs through radical feminist critiques, such as Ferguson's, and mirrors Weber's concerns. However, as was stated earlier in the chapter, organizations are not entities in their own right that 'do things' to people. Organizations are made up of individuals, and it is these individuals who affect others by their actions.

FEMINIST PERSPECTIVES ON ORGANIZATIONS

Organizations are part of society and therefore reflect dominant ideologies within society. Women's position in society is reflected in organizations by the horizontal and vertical gendered division of labour. Hearn & Parkin (1987, pp. 90–91) note that:

In most organisations (gender) divisions of labour are reinforced by (gender) divisions of authority and power, as expressed through hierarchy, and vice versa … In turn hierarchical organisational structures make for hierarchical interpersonal, including sexual, relations between people in organisations.

This gendered hierarchy within organizations is not questioned within classical organizational theory, which is based on the premise that men will hold power and authority in organizations as they do in the private sphere. Management is traditionally viewed as a male trait, and women cannot therefore be managers, or be as successful, simply because they are not male. The gender blindness of classical organizational theory has meant that the study of organizational life is limited. To ignore feminist critiques is to narrow the vision of how we can structure organizations.

Denhardt & Perkins (cited in Ferguson 1984, p. 5) argue, from a feminist perspective, that domination by hierarchies is not essential to the achievement of important goals and actually restricts the growth of the organization and its members.

Activity 11.7

Do you think that it is possible for organizations to be non-hierarchical? Can you think of alternative ways of organizing?

Feminist theories may be useful in giving us a broader understanding of organizational structure. For example, the feminist analysis of patriarchy can help us to understand the workings of male power and control within organizations. However, the biggest impact that feminist critiques of organizations have probably had involves focusing attention on what was invisible in classical theory: the effect of hierarchical relations between people, normally men and women. The clearest example of this is the recognition in recent years of the fairly widespread sexual harassment of women within organizations. Changes in the law have meant that large organizations have clear regulations to deal with this. The effect of sexual harassment on (mainly) women members of organizations can be traumatic, influencing both physical and mental health. This is in turn bad for an organization as staff will not function well in their posts.

Relationships between organizational members are not all abusive. Many people establish personal relationships within the workplace, indicating that the organization is not simply a place of work for its members. However, as Hearn & Parkin (1987) point out, modern organizational life, with its rationalization, is opposed

to this. Organizations can be physically structured in ways to prevent personal relationships forming, as seen, for example, in open space offices where one can be seen at all times.

At this point, it is appropriate to examine some of the issues facing occupational therapists, who are still, in the main, women.

OCCUPATIONAL THERAPISTS AND ORGANIZATIONS

Most occupational therapists work within organizations, although an increasing number are self-employed or freelance therapists. The most conventional areas of work include large agencies such as hospitals and social work departments. Occupational therapists therefore find themselves in the midst of an organization. The aim of this part of the chapter is to explore some of the issues raised above and consider their application and relevance to occupational therapy.

WORKING IN BUREAUCRATIC ORGANIZATIONS

We have already noted how Etzioni described organizations as being social units orientated towards specific goals, and how Weber's work highlights the fact that organizations are often concerned with the business of administration: controlling, managing and coordinating. It is quite clear that most occupational therapists work in bureaucratic organizations that have formal chains of command, clear rules and clear hierarchies. Giddens (1992, p. 135) draws attention to the fact that organizations are formal in nature, including rules, hierarchy of offices and regularized duties that officials perform. This can be clearly identified in a hospital or social services occupational therapy section. The hierarchy often involves occupational therapy assistants, support staff and basic-grade therapists reporting to senior therapists, who in turn report to head occupational therapists. The hierarchy continues, the head of service being responsible to another manager, and so on. Even where occupational therapists are single professionals within a team, they usually have clear managerial and professional line management.

Having established that therapists work in bureaucratic organizations, it is also useful to refer back to some of the problems with bureaucracies. Merton (in Haralambos and Holborn 1995, p. 275) feels that bureaucrats are inflexible in dealing with innovation and improvisation, and are frequently devoted to the rules, emphasizing impersonality. Occupational therapists may thus find themselves confronted with the inflexibility of their manager regarding the implementation of a new treatment procedure or assessment, system of recording notes or approach to their work.

THE PROBLEM OF INFLEXIBILITY

An example of this is the occupational therapist wishing to introduce a new assessment procedure; for example the Canadian Occupational Performance Measure, which would require purchasing the assessment, a longer assessment period with the client/patient and the training of occupational therapy staff in the assessment procedure. The manager may feel that this is unnecessary as the service is meeting its goals without the new assessment and the length of time allocated to the assessment process is already long enough. There may be a stated number of patients/clients required (by the organization) to be seen by the therapist each day. The conflict of the organization's goals, concerned with *quantity* of service, with professional goals, concerned with *quality* of service, is therefore raised in bureaucratic organizations.

The conflict between the organization's policies and the priorities of the professional have been touched on earlier in this chapter in relation to street-level bureaucracy. It is worth exploring this concept further in relation to occupational therapists.

Occupational therapists as street-level bureaucrats

We have already seen how Lipsky (1980) identified that professionals such as social workers often have to bend and shape the rules in order to get the job done. He also identified that work guidelines designed to increase efficiency and client throughput very often conflict with professional values. The example above highlights the tension between the therapist who wants to do a thorough assessment, which can be time-consuming, and the organization, which wants as many people as possible to be seen as quickly as possible within the shortest time by the least number of staff. This conflict is often most apparent for students, who will complain to college lecturers that what they are being taught is idealistic and does not match with the 'real world' that they encounter during fieldwork placement. Graduate therapists also experience this tension; as a result, some leave the profession or take a sideways move into jobs, perhaps with small voluntary organizations, in which they can use their skills but are not as constrained.

Activity 11.8

Have you experienced instances of therapists bending or breaking rules in order to 'get the job done'?

Townsend (1996) carried out an ethnographic study of mental health services in Canada and described how the way in which such services were organized limited practice. She discovered that the therapists' desire to deliver holistic and empowering services was restricted by such things as limitations on the use of petty cash and the overall philosophy of the organization, which stressed psychoeducational approaches rather than real occupations and the rigid structure of programmes. An indication is also given of the way in which therapists deal with the fact that the service is only funded to operate during daytime hours. For example, work schedules may be staggered or time off in lieu may be taken to cover work outside normal hours.

Although the above paints a very negative picture of the working life of a therapist, it is not all doom and gloom. One of the important aspects of work that keeps therapists going is the informal structures present in the workplace.

The importance of informal structures

In contrast to the assumption that the only components of an organization are formal bureaucratic ones, Blau (1974) highlights the importance of unofficial practices within organizations. These form part of the informal processes and are further explained by Giddens (1992) as being informal social relationships, expressive actions, humour and laughter. These processes can again be identified in occupational therapy settings where formal processes, i.e. team briefing, performance appraisal or career review, ward or unit clinical meetings and management meetings, do exist. However, much goes on in informal settings, and the informal communication network often yields interesting and informative information. Lunch, coffee breaks and social get-togethers with staff from within and outside the occupational therapy setting lead to information-sharing and the exchange of ideas as well as humour, relationship-building and informal social interaction. It is even suggested by some sociologists that these informal structures reinforce the solidarity of the organisation (Fine 1992).

Case study 11.1 is a description of a typical 'morning in the life of' an occupational therapist working with cardiac rehabilitation patients following heart surgery in a rehabilitation hospital. After reading it, consider the formal and informal relationships and interactions that she has within her organizational setting. Note what type of interactions they are and how many she engages in the short space of time. Also, reflect on the different types of power discussed earlier in the chapter.

THE CHANGING ORGANIZATIONAL CONTEXT

It is important to consider why it might be relevant for occupational therapists to be aware of organizational structure and bureaucracy. We have already highlighted some of the tensions for therapists of working in a bureaucracy and the importance of informal networks. However, there is some discussion that bureaucracy is on

---

Case study 11.1 A 'morning in the life of' an occupational therapist

Lisa is a Senior II occupational therapist. She arrives at work at 8.30 am and meets with her occupational therapy assistant (OTA) in the occupational therapy (OT) department. She discusses five patients whom she wants the OTA to see that morning, recapping on the aims of the activities to be carried out and highlighting any relevant information gained from the previous morning's ward meeting. The other staff arrive between 8.30 am and 9 am, and Lisa greets them all, catching up on gossip or other interesting news.

Lisa has a second-year OT student with her for 5 weeks, and she asks the student to go with the OTA and observe her for the first hour of the morning. She then goes to the ward. *En route*, she meets the physiotherapist from the ward, and they walk together and discuss Mrs Jones, who requires a home visit that afternoon. Lisa and the physiotherapist are going together, so they arrange times and finalize details. On the way, they make jokes about the anxious new medical student and discuss how they can convince the consultant not to discharge a patient whom they believe is not ready to go home.

On the ward, Lisa meets with the nurse in charge and reminds her that she is seeing two patients for dressing practice and will then be running a relaxation group. Mid-morning, Lisa and the student return to the OT department, where they quickly drink a coffee with the other OT staff and review the morning's work. They remember that they have to telephone the husband of the patient whom they are taking home that afternoon. They do so and then return to the ward for a ward meeting involving the clinical team led by the consultant, Mr Anderson. At the end of the meeting, the team discusses where they will go for a ward administrator's retirement party.

On returning to the OT department, Lisa meets with her head OT to discuss a report that is being prepared for Mr Landrock, the rehabilitation services manager.

---

the decline. It is even suggested that modern organizations are moving towards adhocracy, which is described by Mintzberg (in Haralambos & Holborn 1995, p. 282) as involving innovation, teamwork and ever-shifting relationships on *ad hoc* projects.

Thompson (in Haralambos & Holborn 1995, p. 288) suggests that organizations are changing and that bureaucracies still exist, but that more flexibility and innovative practice is gradually being introduced. Thus, although many organizations are still bureaucratic in nature, there is some debate that they are perhaps becoming more flexible and open to innovation. This runs in parallel with occupational therapy, which, it has been suggested, requires some organization, administration and management, but that innovative practice, teamwork and various *ad hoc* or informal interactions are in concert with the principles of the profession. Some of these changes are highlighted by Gage (1995), who emphasizes the rapidly changing administrative structures of some hospitals in Canada, which also impact on the way in which care is delivered. She notes that while these changes may be disconcerting for therapists used to traditional structures (distinct departments, a clear demarcation of roles, etc.), they can also provide an opportunity to re-engineer services in a more client-driven format.

CONCLUSION

Organizations have a major impact on our lives, either as members of organizations or in their more general effect on our families and communities. Many writers, not least Weber, have been concerned about the effect of bureaucracies on the individuals who come in contact with them, and their effect more widely on our social structure. The concepts of power and control are crucial in understanding the impact that organizations have on their members and clients as well as their internal structures.

Understanding organizations, their structure and their workings can give the occupational therapist an overall perspective on the institution in which they find themselves working. This knowledge can help therapists in determining the type of organization within which they work. A clear understanding of the organizational and management structure facilitates awareness of the lines of management and the communication procedures within the organization. An appreciation of the limitations and advantages of the specific organizational structure and the goals of that organization aids the therapists in ensuring that they can either work within the ethos of that organization or help to change it.

REFERENCES

Blau P 1956 Bureaucracy in modern society. Random House, New York
Blau P M 1974 On the nature of organisations. John Wiley, New York
Blau P, Schoenherr R A 1971 The structure of organisations. Basic Books, New York
Blau P, Scott W 1963 Formal organisations: a comparative approach. Routledge & Kegan Paul, London
Braverman H 1974 Labor and monopoly, capital. Monthly Review Press, New York
Burns T, Stalker G 1961 The management of innovation. Tavistock, London
Caplow T 1964 Principles of organisation. Harcourt Brace, London
Clegg S 1979 The theory of power and organisation. Routledge & Kegan Paul, London
Crozier M 1964 The bureaucratic phenomenon. University of Chicago Press, Chicago
Eldridge J, Crombie A 1974 A sociology of organisations. George Allen & Unwin, Oxford
Eldridge J (ed.) (1971) Max Weber: the interpretation of social reality. Nelson, London
Etzioni A 1964 Modern organisations. Prentice Hall, Englewood Cliffs, NJ
Ferguson K 1984 The feminist case against bureaucracy. Temple University Press, Philadelphia

Fine G A 1992 Letting off steam? Redefining a restaurant work environment. In: Giddens A (ed.) 1992 Human societies. Polity Press: Blackwell, Oxford
French J, Raven B 1959 The bases of social power. In: Cartwright D (ed.) Studies in social power. University of Michigan Press, Ann Arbor
Gage M 1995 Re-engineering of health care: opportunity or threat for occupational therapists? Canadian Journal of Occupational Therapy 62(4): 197–207
Galbraith J K 1972 The new industrial estate, 2nd edn. Pelican, Harmondsworth
Gerth H, Mills C W 1948 Max Weber: essays in sociology. Routledge & Kegan Paul, London
Gouldner A 1954 Patterns of industrial bureaucracy. Free Press, New York
Hall R 1972 Organisations: structure and processes and outcomes. Prentice Hall, Englewood Cliffs, NJ
Handy C 1993 Understanding organisations, 4th edn. Penguin, London
Haralambos M (ed.) 1989 Developments in sociology, vol. 5. Causeway Press, Ormskirk
Haralambos M, Holborn M 1995 Sociology. Themes and perspectives, 4th edn. Collins Educational, London
Hearn J, Parkin W 1987 'Sex' at 'work': the power and paradox of organisation sexuality. Wheatsheaf, Brighton

Lipsky M 1980 Street level bureaucracy: dilemas of the individual in public services. Russell Sage Foundation, NY

Lockwood D 1956 The black coated worker. Allen & Unwin, London

Mayer J 1956 Max Weber and German politics. Faber & Faber, London

Merton R 1952 Bureaucratic structure and personality. In: Merton R (ed.) Reader in bureaucracy. Free Press, Glencoe

Michels R 1921 Political parties. Free Press, Chicago

Parkinson C N 1958 Parkinson's law. John Murray, London

Parsons T (1960) Structure and process in modern societies. Free Press, New York

Peter L, Hull R 1969 The Peter principle. Souvenir Press, London

Salaman G 1979 Work organisations: resistance and control. Longman, London

Sofer C 1972 Organisations in theory and practice. Heinemann, London

Townsend E 1996 Enabling empowerment: using simulations versus real occupations. Canadian Journal of Occupational Therapy 63(2): 114–127

12

The sociology of the health professions

R. K. Jones   Averil Stewart

SOCIOLOGICAL STUDY OF THE PROFESSIONS

In everyday language, it is commonplace to designate a variety of occupations, such as teaching, nursing and occupational therapy, as professions. More and more occupations are now adopting for themselves the title of profession in order to suggest a certain quality of service ('professional carpet-fitter') or to distinguish themselves from people who undertake the same activity as a hobby (e.g. 'professional footballer'). Traditionally, however, the professions were taken to mean lawyers, doctors, clerics and officers in the armed forces.

Activity 12.1

Make a list of those occupations which refer to themselves as professions.

The sociological approach to the study of the professions can be roughly divided into two branches:

- the more functionalist approach, with its focus on identifying the characteristics of a profession
- conflict- and interactionist-influenced approaches, which are more interested in how occupations attain the status of profession, in the behaviour of professionals and in the nature of the power they wield.

An understanding of the insights from the latter

approaches in particular will help the professional to keep uppermost in her or his mind the question, 'Am I, as a professional, acting in my own interests or those of my client?' First, however let us consider the traditional approach.

A FUNCTIONALIST PERSPECTIVE

From a functionalist perspective, the existence of professions is a way of organizing particular occupations that reflects the socially important nature of their work. These occupations are involved in the application of specialist knowledge that is only available through lengthy training courses and is widely accepted as involving values that reflect the common good. The higher financial rewards of the professions are justified by the need for lengthy training during which the student is less well off. The autonomy and control over their own affairs that society allows the professions also reflect a kind of bargain by which the professions guarantee the community the maintenance of high standards of service in return for such freedoms. Parsons called this 'common sense' view of the professions, a view that the professions typically hold of themselves, 'cognitive rationality' (1951). Thus the traditional usage of the word 'profession' elicits some notion of service and actions on the part of the professional that are driven first and foremost by the client's interests, rather than by the financial interests of the professional.

Carr-Saunders, writing in 1925 (quoted in Volmer & Mills 1966), suggested that 'A profession may perhaps be defined as an occupation based upon specialised intellectual study and training, the purpose of which is to supply skilled service or advice to others for a definite fee or salary.' It is obvious that this is much too wide a definition, in that it lumps together a variety of disparate occupations that share little in common. This definition could include occupations as different as, for example, a consultant computer analyst and a medical consultant. The inventory or trait approach to the problem of definition is an attempt more clearly to delineate occupations falling under the category of profession.

Trait approach

Greenwood (1957) proposed a list of traits or characteristics that he identified as distinguishing a profession:

- a systematic body of theory
- authority
- a restriction of admission
- a code of ethics
- a professional culture.

Activity 12.2
To what extent does occupational therapy possess the characteristics described by Greenwood?

Millerson (1964) took a similar approach and identified three traits commonly cited in the literature:

- adherence to a code of professional conduct
- organization
- a skill-based theoretical knowledge.

The trait approach has particular benefits. It has allowed us to characterize those occupations which are developing particular levels of skill and organization in some ways comparable with the established professions. These occupations, such as nursing, social work, physiotherapy and occupational therapy, are called 'semiprofessions' because they lack one or more of the inventory elements. Semiprofessional status is seen to be a reflection of the weak development of a systematic body of theoretical knowledge, compared with a stronger basis in specific methods of working, and the development of specific professional values such as service orientation.

Attempts of this nature to define professions could be criticized on a number of points:

1. These lists contain characteristics that the so-called professions would like to see themselves as possessing. It could be argued that the 'socially important' tasks and values pursued by the professions are not necessarily perceived as important by all sections of society.

2. Questions can be raised of whether the professions are necessarily devoted to pursuing

---

Activity 12.3

Can you give any examples from your experience of interprofessional conflict? How was the conflict resolved?

---

the community interest rather than their own. If all the professions are involved in the pursuit of the public interest and are based on broadly held values, how is it that conflicts arise between different professional groups?

3. It is not clear that the status of professionals is related to either the degree or the complexity of the task involved. Many professionals depend as much on interpersonal skills as on the command of a systematic body of knowledge.

In summary, the functionalist approach fails to indicate how certain occupations achieve or seek to achieve professional status in a historical context, and how this professional status is maintained. To overcome these weaknesses, any analysis of the professions must be linked with the processes at work in the larger society.

A CONFLICT PERSPECTIVE

George Bernard Shaw (1906) once famously stated that 'all professions are conspiracies against the laity'. This distinction between the professions and others is taken up by O'Donnell (1981), who notes, 'The difference between the professions and other occupations is that they have succeeded in convincing the public of their special skills and importance of their need for corresponding privileges, whereas others have not.' There is thus a perspective that sees the professions as engaged in a power struggle with other sections of society.

A Marxist perspective

In countries with health-care systems, such as Britain, the state employs most health-care professionals directly via the National Health Service. Conflict arises in the employer–employee nature of this relationship, just as with any other occupational group, in terms of pay and conditions, although negotiation is sometimes with professional associations rather than trade unions. In privatized health-care systems (such as that of the USA), the professional is to an even greater extent subject to corporate control.

Some sociologists have argued that being employed by bureaucracies necessitates conflict between administrators and professionals, resulting in a fragmented and alienated professional body. Moreover, the managers are seen increasingly to be winning this conflict, as a capitalist system demands a high division of labour and the routinization of activity in order to keep down costs. In effect, professionals become simply well-paid labour. This process by which professions lose their power and autonomy is called 'proletarianization' (Braverman 1974).

The notion of the proletarianization of health-care professionals reflects the broader Marxist analysis of medicine. From this perspective, health care is seen as becoming a commodity to be bought and sold just like any other. Profit-making drug companies and insurance companies, for example, use their powerful influence to direct the nature of health care (Navarro 1986).

Criticisms of the Marxist approach have been that:

- it overstates the case for the deskilling of professionals – in some areas, professional practice is becoming even more skilled rather than more routine
- it underestimates the positive role of health care in contemporary capitalist societies – it is not just about keeping the labour force well enough to continue being exploited
- it does not deal with male domination within the professions
- it does not get to grips with the dynamics of the professional–client interaction.

AN ACTION PERSPECTIVE

By the mid-1960s and early 70s, the study of the professions was quite clearly moving towards an 'action' approach. This perspective had its roots in Weberian sociology and the focus on the meanings that people attach to situations and their subsequent consequences. Studies by Becker and others were the outcome of a tradition that took as its subject matter the actions and interactions of groups, how they constituted their social world as participants and how they constructed their careers. The professional principles of altruism, service and high ethical standards were therefore seen as aspects of the day-to-day world within which experts lived and worked. In the study *Boys in white* (Becker et al 1961), trainee physicians were portrayed as developing over the course of their training, cynicism and pragmatism rather than altruism and idealism.

Sociologists within this tradition (e.g. Hughes 1963) were interested in why some occupational groups but not others managed to be designated as professions, or to put it another way, how professions managed to persuade society that they deserved a privileged position. The notion of a 'professional project' to describe this process was another concept originating from the symbolic interactionist tradition (MacDonald 1995).

The concern with the manner in which groups of people act in order to acquire the characteristics of a profession and how they negotiate and maintain their positions of power and autonomy in society is a feature of the work of Elston (1991), Friedson (1970) and Larson (1977).

Power and autonomy in the professions

Power relations between the professions have increased with the expansion of the public sector. It is commonly assumed that higher professionals such as doctors, dentists and lawyers are in a stronger market position than lower professionals such as teachers, nurses and occupational therapists. Most recent studies are at pains to show how they attained their autonomy and how they dominate related occupations. Furthermore, such autonomy excludes external interference and criticism. One important aspect that is considered is whether the professions exercise sufficient control over their members.

Elston (1991) demarcates three kinds of professional autonomy:

- political autonomy – the mandate to make policy decisions in their field
- economic autonomy – the right to set their own remuneration
- clinical autonomy – to establish standards and control of clinical performance.

Activity 12.4

To what extent does occupational therapy demonstrate the kinds of autonomy described in the text?

Friedson: professional closure and the control of related professions

The term 'professional closure' relates to the way in which an occupational group is able to control entry to itself. Friedson (1970) pointed out that medicine not only secured its own autonomy, but could also regulate the tasks and boundaries of nursing and other allied occupations. He highlighted three key elements:

1. Professional autonomy depends on state power and a sponsoring élite with the provision of a licence to practise legitimating the title of profession
2. Professional autonomy is the result of a power struggle, which emerges independently of the sponsoring élite; it requires the approval of a broader section of society
3. The professions' cognitive and normative features (which are part of the characteristics used to define them) are not static. For example, the content of curricula in occupational therapy has changed drastically over the years.

Professional dominance in practice is exemplified by Larkin's (1980) study of the way in which dentists controlled dental dressers, doing so for their own self-interests rather than for any

---

Activity 12.5

To what extent is occupational therapy regulated by doctors?

---

altruistic motive. In Britain, the British Dental Association pressured the Ministry of Health to make it illegal for dental dressers to either diagnose or carry out elementary routine surgical procedures.

Another aspect of the professional autonomy entails the notion of knowledge as power (Foucault 1980, Jones 1975). Several writers have stressed that knowledge is a core trait of professionalization (e.g. Abbott 1988). Knowledge as we know it today could not have emerged in earlier society as it was then tied to well-established social institutions such as the Church and academia. Today, it is tied up with the empirical world of nature (MacDonald 1995), subject to wider scrutiny and demands for evidence.

A clear sociological analysis of professional knowledge is to be found in a number of studies. Nettleton (1992), for example, sees modern dentistry as emerging out of the reconstitution of knowledge and its focus on the mouth as object. Thus there is now a whole body of theory, practices and professional jargon, developed largely in the twentieth century, in relation to one small part of the body. Arney's (1983) study of the rise of modern technology and its use in obstetrics shows how this has resulted in greater medical control. Midwifery not only has been relegated to a subordinate position, but in North America has virtually ceased to exist.

Larson and the professional market

For Larson (1977), professionalization is an attempt to translate one order of scarce resources – special knowledge and skills – into another, that of social and economic rewards. To maintain scarcity implies a tendency to monopoly: monopoly of expertise in the market and monopoly of prestige in the stratification system. The focus on the constitution of professional markets leads to comparing different professions in terms of the marketability of their specific 'cognitive resources'. It therefore leads to the exclusion of professions such as the military and the clergy, which do not transact their services on the market. The focus on collective social mobility accentuates the

relationships that professions form with different systems of social stratification, in particular accentuating the role that educational systems play in different structures of social inequality.

It follows from what has been said that one way to analyse the actions of professions is in terms of attempts to protect their market position, that is to say, to what extent professions attempt to prevent other occupations trying to 'muscle in' on their patch.

Activity 12.6

Does occupational therapy have any specific cognitive resource that it can market?
  Does the profession attempt to protect its 'market'?

WOMEN AND THE PROFESSIONS

Women have been subject to patriarchal domination within the health professions as in other areas of social life. The historical demarcation of tasks considered appropriate for women has carried over into the work situation in the guise of caring. The notion of social closure is applied to groups excluding others access to rewards (Parkin 1974). The consequences of the development of nursing and social work, for example, minimized academic or esoteric knowledge and placed considerable importance on empathy, love and caring for others.

The growth of a profession demonstrates, in the early stages, considerable contention for a stake in the power struggle (Jones 1985). Predominantly female occupations such as occupational therapy and nursing must constantly resist patriarchal advances. Midwifery is a good example of aspiring medical practitioners taking over the role of the traditional midwife in order to gain access to health treatment and therefore professional dominance of the household (Marland 1993).

With the transfer of healing from women to men, medical practice was relocated from the domestic or household arena to that of the market. This sounded the death knell for women's participation in healing practices. Witz (1992) explored the gendered nature of occupational

---

Box 12.1 Strategies for occupational closure
(Witz 1992)

- *Exclusionary strategies*: An occupation decides criteria for membership based on existing membership and qualifications. The existing members 'fix' the rules so that only people like them can get in

- *Demarcationary strategies*: Boundaries are drawn between the dominant and subordinate occupations, for example medicine and occupational therapy, laying out what are accepted areas of practice

- *Inclusionary strategies*: This refers to how excluded groups, for example women, devise strategies for access to the powerful groups

- *Dual closure strategies*: This refers to the process by which the excluded establish their own occupational field

---

Activity 12.7

The fact that occupational therapy is a largely female profession has been regarded as a reason for its lack of professional status. How true is this?

---

strategies, identifying that as the agents are men or women, gender may form the basis of solidarity. Strategies for occupational closure are located in patriarchal structures and manifest themselves as shown in Box 12.1.

The challenge from women to the health-care system has been on two fronts: the way in which it is practised, and the place of women within it. This has been one element of the increasing challenge to the medical profession.

EROSION OF MEDICAL DOMINANCE

In recent years, several sociologists have indicated that, although the medical profession has enjoyed considerable power, this is being challenged in a number of areas (Gabe et al 1994, Samson 1995).

One major challenge to the health professions arises from the growing strength of the power of managers and administrators within health services. This process is referred to as managerialism, and it has been particularly noticeable

in Britain since the introduction of the NHS management reforms following the Griffiths report of 1983. Further changes within the UK health system, with the introduction of the internal market and its split between purchasers and providers, have weakened hospital professionals in particular and seen the introduction of business managers into general practice. This process would seem to support the notion of proletarianization discussed earlier.

Further challenges to the established medical dominance have come from a number of sources. The rise of the new nursing élite has begun a process of redefining the relationship between medicine and nursing, with an inclination towards the role of nurse practitioners backed up by the development of Departments of Nursing in higher education. Also, alternative and complementary therapies have seen their number of consultations increase as people now have an alternative to the biomedical approaches, which have little to offer people with chronic illnesses (Saks 1994). At the same time, increasing numbers of self-help groups have given patients a collective voice with which to challenge the professionals.

Challenges have also increased in the form of patients seeking recourse to litigation when dissatisfied with medical treatment (Dingwall 1994). This may have been helped by the fact that the public has greater access to perspectives critical of biomedicine and of the professions through popular medical journalism and other forms of media coverage (Bury & Gabe 1994).

OCCUPATIONAL THERAPY AS A PROFESSION

Examination of the sociological literature on the professions opens a number of avenues that bear investigation. Some of these avenues are of plain interest, whereas others raise crucial questions regarding the very nature of the way in which occupational therapy is practised. This section of the chapter looks at:

- the professional characteristics of

occupational therapy and the extent to which it can lay claim to the status of profession
- the professional socialization of students
- the current context of practice.

PROFESSIONAL CHARACTERISTICS OF OCCUPATIONAL THERAPY

If we were to look at occupational therapy from a functionalist perspective, we would want to look at the extent to which it contains the characteristics of a profession. We might wish to investigate the extent to which it meets the traits identified by Greenwood (see above). This next section will give you the opportunity to reflect on the answers you gave in Activity 12.1.

Systematic body of theory

There is considerable evidence from educational programmes of how occupational therapists acquire a range of knowledge and skills, much of which is, however, drawn from other disciplines and was until recently based largely on a medical model. Core elements of the curriculum are also drawn from the behavioural and social sciences. Moreover, curriculum content, in its totality, is not consistent across the UK, far less across countries and continents, and there is increasingly an overlap with other health-care groups. This can be advantageous in terms of cooperation and professional groupings in higher education, but it also destroys the argument of there being a unique base of specialized knowledge. It is not surprising therefore that a lack in this key area has resulted in the designation of occupational therapy as a semiprofession. This status is also reflected in the attitudes of the established professionals. A report in the *Times Higher Educational Supplement* (Utley 1996) referred to one academic who spoke of the 'mums army of PAMs' (professions allied to medicine). However, in terms of the development of a systematic body of theory, moves have been made in this direction with the development of the Model of Human Occupation, the Canadian Model of Occupational Performance and the discipline of occupational science.

Authority

Occupational therapists have historically had little authority. In Britain, for example, referrals have been filtered by doctors or social workers, and until relatively recently occupational therapists were not able to prescribe wheelchairs without a doctor's signature. This lack of authority is reflected in the title 'professions *Supplementary* (or allied) to medicine' which is shared with physiotherapists and others. In some respects, this lack of authority is changing, and therapists are attaining more autonomy in a number of areas. However, they are simultaneously losing it in others. We have already noted the idea of proletarianization, and this can perhaps be seen in the fact that many occupational therapists are now managed by generic managers rather than someone from their own profession.

Craik (1995) in Britain and Yerxa (1995) in America have identified the importance of the issue of control of the profession. They see some of the challenges to the profession coming from:

- drives towards 'generic' therapists
- a focus on technical training rather than reflective education
- a lack of understanding of the multidimensional nature of occupational therapy
- the relative youth and therefore autonomy of the profession.

Restriction of admission

Yates (1996), in her Casson Memorial Lecture at the College of Occupational Therapists annual conference, highlighted how, in the past, admission policies and funding arrangements in Britain discriminated against people on low incomes, men and mature married females. She also emphasized how, despite increases in the population of people from ethnic minority backgrounds, these communities are still under-represented in the profession. Thus restriction of admission to the profession has existed in the past as deliberate policy – in the 1960s men were not accepted into at least six of the training schools –

or continues to exist for broader structural reasons. By this we mean that, despite the apparent growth in higher education, people from ethnic minorities and low-income backgrounds, and disabled people, are underrepresented in this sector of education.

Attempts to redress the balance and make the profession more representative of the population as a whole have been made and will continue. These changes have been driven by an increasing awareness of equal opportunities issues, although Yates (1996) suggests that the profession still has much work to do and is perhaps not as advanced as it likes to believe.

Code of ethics

The code of conduct contains a number of moral issues, such as 'treating the client with respect', that are common to other health- and social care professions. There are also components that prescribe behaviour in relation to advertising and the acceptance of gifts, to name but two examples. Failure to adhere to the professional code by, for example, indulging in inappropriate sexual activity could, in Britain, lead to being guilty of infamous conduct and being struck off the register set up by the Professions Supplementary to Medicine (PSM) Act of 1960.

Activity 12.8

One of the criticisms of professions is that they 'look after their own' and that transgressors are rarely punished.

Find your professional association's code of conduct. Is there a record of cases that have been in breach of the code? Have you witnessed any breach of code or spirit of the code? What should be done if a colleague is perceived as being incompetent?

Professional culture

Occupational therapy would seem to have a strong professional culture. This can be seen in the existence of a shared set of beliefs and values that are articulated in the various journals of the profession. It is also obvious in smaller ways: in the wearing of professional badges, and other signs of allegiance such as car stickers, T-shirts, etc. The acquisition of this professional culture takes place during the education of new therapists through a process of socialization.

PROFESSIONAL SOCIALIZATION

From a functionalist perspective, the education and training of occupational therapists represents a form of secondary socialization during which students learn their new role and its associated norms and values. While any new cohort of selected and self-selected students will have wide ranging life experiences, there is nevertheless a common commitment to and awareness of the profession and the career they have chosen to follow. Add to this the common expectations of lecturers and later fieldwork educators, and the process of socializing new recruits into the profession begins to take shape. New knowledge and skills are imparted and developed, but perhaps even more fundamental are the examples, attitudes and relationships that develop between students and staff. Are these relationships authoritarian and powerful or based on mutual respect, negotiation and cooperation, in pursuit of a mutual goal, that of becoming competent to practise as an occupational therapist? In other words, professional values are instilled not only in an explicit way through lectures, but also by implication. How students are treated and empowered, or otherwise, can influence the approaches they subsequently adopt with their future clients.

However, as we have seen in Chapter 2, the functionalist perspective has been criticized for presenting an 'oversocialized' view of people. Symbolic interactionists such as Goffman have identified the way in which people 'play' with roles in order to create an impression.

Activity 12.9

To what extent have you or are you being transformed into an occupational therapist, or do you sometimes tell tutors what you think they want to hear, or behave in ways you believe will be approved of by each individual fieldwork educator?

Not only is a professional identity established early on, but so too are differences between one profession and another, albeit at a simplistic and potentially stereotypical level. These may be exaggerated in the early days in order to create a sense of professional identity and loyalty, resulting in a rigid demarcation that prevents interprofessional cooperation at a later stage. Attempts to promote shared learning and working on projects of mutual interest and relevance can be influential in avoiding this danger. Currently, two undergraduate programmes (the University of East Anglia and the University of Southampton) in the UK for occupational therapists and physiotherapists share large components of the curriculum, relating to communication skills, management and research. The outcomes from longitudinal evaluations are eagerly awaited in order to ascertain the level of cooperation and awareness of each other's roles compared with those students who progress through educational vocational programmes with less interprofessional contact.

Activity 12.10

Make a list of all the aspects of occupational therapy that you think make it different from other health-care professions. How do you learn about differences between health-care professions?

What is your attitude to other professional groups and from where did that attitude come?

CURRENT CONTEXT OF PRACTICE

As we have noted, various forces are weakening the power and autonomy of professions. Three important issues to consider are:

- the development of competency-based training programmes for therapists
- the rise of managerialism
- the disability movement.

Developments in education and training

It could be argued that, until recently, the professions, in collaboration with higher education institutions, identified the knowledge and skills that were required by employers in health care and by society in general (Barnett 1994). There is now, however, increasing evidence that employers are identifying the competencies that they wish to purchase (Yerxa 1995). In Britain, their demands are being met through alternative routes for people to gain qualifications such as National/Scottish Vocational Qualifications (N/SVQs). As a result, there are new tensions between professions and prospective employers. These can either be seen as threats leading to greater entrenchment or as opportunities that look for ways of harmonizing what might be seen as incompatible and competing forces.

In the past, it has been the content of courses and their assessment procedures that have been criticized in judgments about professional competency. The emphasis is now on the actual outcomes, which may be reached by a variety of routes, from traditional full-time courses, to distance learning with credit being given for prior learning and relevant experience, or to work-based learning and the assessment of actual observable behaviours. Depending on the nature and complexity of the job, evidence may be sought of the candidate's underpinning knowledge that contributes to the competence. This evidence may also give confidence of the individual's ability to respond in similar or more complex situations with and without supervision. As such, this is a rather different approach to establishing competence in a range of tasks, compared with conventional programmes of study. This may, of course, have implications for the socialization of new recruits.

Managerialism

As we have noted, the professions are increasingly subject to having their agenda set by managers and are losing power and autonomy in the process. An indication of this is the increased demand for more skill mix, which could be a short step on the road to generic professions. Is this such a bad thing if we remind ourselves of the question at the start of the chapter – Whose interests do I serve: the client's or the profession's?'

Variations can be anathema to some professional groups. In the same way, the concept of 'skill mix' in the workforce is viewed by some as a cheap option for employers before any evaluative measures have been established. Skill mix can enable the specific skills of each member to be harnessed, resulting in greater efficiency and personal satisfaction, but getting the right mix depends on flexibility. Support staff can help to reduce waiting lists by being delegated appropriate tasks for which they have been trained. To take this a step further, and in recognition of the client as the expert with regard to his own condition, self-assessment can be a tool that reduces demands on professionals' time and focuses attention onto personal control and choice. On the other hand, changes may be made in order to meet short-term financial targets under the guise of providing more focused patient care.

Another element of the new managerialism is the increased demand for outcome measures, cost-effectiveness and clinical audit (de Clive-Lowe 1996). Of course, it is important to know that our interventions are effective, but it is also important to remember that what is a good outcome for the client may not be recognized as a valid outcome by the agency that provides the funds. Where the client him or herself is the funding agent, this puts events in a different light. At this point, it is important to consider the perspective of the disability movement.

The disability movement

The increasingly powerful voice of the disability movement should cause occupational therapists and other professionals to reflect on their practice. According to one anecdote, a disabled person was heard to remark that disabled people have traditionally been little more than job creation schemes for professionals. Thus professionals have sought to maintain their position by keeping disabled people dependent, despite claims to enable and empower. This approach is reflected in an article by Abberley (1995), who suggests that the way in which occupational therapists practise, focusing on the individual, fails to get to grips with the social limitations on people's function. He suggests that where therapeutic intervention fails, this is often put down to the client, and that when there is success, it is claimed to result from modification of the client's perspective by the skill of the therapist.

It has to be said that these findings are based on interviews with only 16 occupational therapists. However, if Abberley's findings are representative, this is something about which the profession needs to be concerned. In a Canadian context, Sherr Klein (1995) has recounted some of her positive and negative contacts with occupational therapy. She calls upon therapists to be allies as well as partners in the struggles that disabled people face in order to take their place in the world (Box 12.2).

Box 12.2 An ally as well as a partner in practice (Sherr Klein 1995)

When I was discharged from hospital the occupational therapists dealt with any necessary adaptations to the house, like banisters and grab bars. What they did not prepare me for was how to live as a disabled person in a world which is not disability friendly. Because I had no role models or friends with disabilities and the rehabilitation professionals had not exposed me to any of the disability organisations, I had the feeling that I was the first person in the world to be going through what I was going through. We need regular checking-in: what do you want? The answer keeps changing, and that is appropriate, but so should the therapy change. We want to collaborate about our programmes and to be partners in the planning and the process.

Without getting complacent, one could challenge Abberley's charges by pointing out that occupational therapists are beginning to address the need to change the wider society rather than just focus on the individual. Townsend (1993), for example, called for the profession to develop its 'social vision' and acknowledge that people are not dependent or independent but interdependent. This perspective is taken up by Grady (1994), who challenges us to:

- review ideas about disability
- work with communities to be more accepting of diversity
- expand our ideas about the role of the wider

environment on the opportunities for disabled people
- consider strategies for expanding choice and inclusion in society
- examine the meaning of community.

The influence of the disability movement of practice is explored further in Chapter 15.

CONCLUSION

The study of the sociology of professions raises a number of questions. It helps us to analyse our position in the health-care 'market' and examine our relationship with our clients. We have highlighted how occupational therapists exist within a complex web of power relationships and how the power of the medical profession is likely to be lessened. Collaborative planning, quality audits and total quality management will play an increasing part in professional practice. Performance measures and professional updating will become a way of life for those who want to survive. Without a reliable measure of the efficacy of professional activities, we could become peripheral, marginalized or perhaps even extinct.

This brave new world is frightening for it almost ignores the client. Bureaucratic, power-driven mechanisms can take away from the humanity of the therapist. At the end of the day, a balance has to be struck that allows for the integrity of the therapist, is flexible to the demands of the organization in economic and political terms but, most importantly of all, meets the needs of consumers, helping to maintain and restore their health and desired way of life.

To conclude this chapter, consider the following questions facing health-care professionals, highlighted by Young (1995):

- Are they willing to share power with patients/clients in a more equal way?
- Are they going to value being members of a profession for what they can offer, rather than the status (power) it gives them?
- What new sources of power can they develop in order to enhance the achievement of agreed organizational goals?

REFERENCES

Abberley P 1995 Disabling ideology in health and welfare – the case of occupational therapy. Disability and Society 10(2): 221–232

Abbott A 1988 The system of professions. University of Chicago Press, London

Arney W R 1983 Power and the profession of obstetrics. University of Chicago Press, London

Barnett R 1994 Limits of competence: knowledge, higher education and society. Open University Press, Milton Keynes

Becker H S, Greer B, Hughes E C, Strauss A L 1961 Boys in white. University of Chicago Press, Chicago.

Braverman H 1974 Labour and monopoly capital: the degradation of work in the twentieth century. Monthly Review Press, New York

Bury M, Gabe J 1994 Television and medicine: medical dominance or trial by media? In: Gabe J, Kelleher D, Williams G (eds) Challenging medicine. Routledge, London

Craik C 1995 Stakeholders in the future of occupational therapy. British Journal of Occupational Therapy 58(12): 517–518

de Clive-Lowe S 1996 Outcome measurement, cost-effectiveness and clinical audit: the importance of standardised assessment to occupational therapists in meeting these new demands. British Journal of Occupational Therapy 59(8): 357–362

Dingwall R 1994 Litigation and the threat to medicine. In: Gabe J, Kelleher D, Williams G (eds) Challenging medicine. Routledge, London

Elston M A 1991 The politics of professional power: medicine in a changing society. In: Gabe J, Calnan M, Bury M (eds) The sociology of the health service: Routledge, London.

Foucault M 1980 Power/knowledge. Harvester Press, Brighton

Friedson E 1970 The profession of medicine. Dodd Mead, New York

Gabe J, Kelleher D, Williams G (eds) 1994 Challenging medicine. Routledge, London

Grady A P 1994 Eleanor Clarke Slagle lecture: building inclusive community: a challenge for occupational therapy. American Journal of Occupational Therapy 49(4): 300–310

Greenwood E 1957 Attributes of a profession. Social Work 2(3): 44–55

Hughes E C 1963 Professions. Daedalus 92:

Jones R K 1975 Knowledge as power. In: Richardson K, Houghton V (eds) Recurrent education. Ward Lock, London

Jones R K (ed) 1985 Sickness and sectarianism. Gower, Aldershot

Klein B, Sherr 1995 An ally as well as a partner in practice. Canadian Journal of Occupational Therapy 62(5): 283–285

Larkin G 1980 Professionalism, dentistry and public health. Social Science and Medicine 14: 223–229

Larson M S 1977 The rise of professionalism: a sociological analysis. University of California Press, London

MacDonald K M 1995 The sociology of the professions. Sage, London

Marland H 1993 The art of midwifery: early modern midwives in Europe. Routledge, New York

Millerson G 1964 The qualifying associations: a study of professionalisation. Routledge, London

Navarro V 1986 Crisis, health and medicine: a social critique. Tavistock, London

Nettleton S 1992 Power, pain and dentistry. Open University Press, Buckingham

O'Donnell M A 1981 A new introduction to sociology. Nelson, London

Parkin F 1974 Strategies of social closure and class formation. In: Parkin F (ed.) The social analysis of class struggle. Tavistock, London.

Parsons T 1951 The social system. Free Press, Glencoe

Saks M 1994 The alternative to medicine. In: Gabe J, Kelleher D, Williams G (eds) 1994 Challenging medicine. Routledge, London

Samson C 1995 The fracturing of medical dominance in British psychiatry. Sociology of Health and Illness 17(2): 245–268

Shaw G B 1906 The doctor's dilemma. Citation in: Partington A (ed.) 1992 The Oxford Dictionary of Quotations (4th edn). Oxford University Press, Oxford, p. 636

Townsend E 1993 Murial Driver Lecture: Occupational therapy's social vision. Canadian Journal of Occupational Therapy 60(4): 174–183

Utley A 1996 Government tightens control of the professions. Times Higher Educational Supplement June 14, p. 6

Volmer H, Mills D L (eds) 1966 Professionalisation. Prentice Hall, New Jersey

Witz A 1992 Professions and patriarchy. Routledge, London

Yates E J 1996 The Casson Memorial Lecture 1996: Equalising opportunities. British Journal of Occupational Therapy 59(8): 352–356

Yerxa E J 1995 Who is the keeper of occupational therapy's practice and knowledge? American Journal of Occupational Therapy 49(4): 295–299

Young A 1995 The politics of professional power in today's health-care market. British Journal of Therapy and Rehabilitation 2(10): 562–565

13

Work

C. Yuill   I. McMillan

THE IMPORTANCE OF WORK

Work is without doubt a very important feature of our lives. From work, we draw not only an income with which to maintain a certain standard of existence, but also social contacts, status and a structure to our lives. Work is something that is regarded positively within most societies and something without which those societies themselves could not exist. But work is not a uniform experience around the globe. It is often bound in with a particular society with differences in attitudes to work existing between different cultures. Work is also highly contradictory. Even though it is something we actively seek in our lives, it is also a source of boredom and frustration. The nature of work itself is also changing. Patterns of employment are undergoing deep transformations, whether on a general scale or between groups within society.

This chapter will seek to explore:

- what work is and why we engage in it
- differences in the experience of work
- sociological theories that explain the existence of work
- changes in patterns of work, namely long-term unemployment
- gender differences in work
- the implications of these issues for occupational therapists.

WHAT IS WORK?

Trying to answer what may seem the rather

pedantic question 'What is work?' is actually a fairly complex task. Work describes a vast range of activities and tasks in our society and can often mean quite different things. When we refer to 'work', we usually mean paid industrial or commercial work, in a factory, hospital or office setting. However, this definition denies a whole range of tasks, activities and occupations that are, in many ways, work. For example, you, the reader, are probably regarding reading this chapters as work, but your perception and experience of the work relating to this chapter will be quite different from that of myself, the author. For a start, you will not be receiving any payment for what you are doing. Secondly, my experience of writing this chapter was bound into a regulated working schedule that started at 9 in the morning and officially finished at 5 in the evening, while you could be reading this chapter during the day or at 4 in the morning as you quote a few references to complete an assignment.

Other people's experience and idea of what work involves could be quite sharply different from those which have been examined above. Someone who has spent 2 weeks on an oil rig or packed in five evenings' overtime in the office, or a mother who rushes home from her part-time job to cook a meal for her children and husband, may not regard reading or writing a chapter in a book as work at all. It could be more akin to what they may regard as a leisure activity.

From this brief discussion of work, you may now see it as something that is quite problematic to define. Basically, work is a highly variable entity that takes on different meanings depending on the social context and the meanings assigned to it by these involved. In reviewing the sociological literature on work, Grint (1991) defined work as 'a socially constructed phenomenon without fixed or universal meanings across space and time'.

Once again, we come across the important concept of the social construction of reality, which has already been highlighted in other chapters, for example in relation to sex and gender, and health and illness. Further complexities of what constitutes work will be discussed throughout this chapter, especially in relation to cultural and gender differences.

Culture and work

The concept of work is bound and constructed by the society within which it takes place. As you will have noticed, definitions of work are quite fluid, and a society's particular culture also influences patterns and arrangements of work. Had this book been published 20 years ago, there would have been an emphasis on Sahlin's (1972) observations of Australian Aboriginal people's attitudes to work. Owing to the availability of nuts, berries and other wild foods, the particular people of his study would only engage in a few hours' activity per day that was classified as 'work', the remaining time being spent talking, meeting friends and with families. However, such cultures are relatively scarce today as a result of the expansion of global Western-style capitalism. This does not mean that each society and culture is becoming a carbon copy of the USA or UK: variation still exists. Japanese working practices provide an interesting example of this. The Western emphasis on competitive individualism is not as apparent in Japanese work. Instead, work is more collectively orientated, emphasis being placed on the group of workers of which one is part. This group is referred to as the *Uchi* ('us'). Not pulling one's weight or letting the group down meets with strong disapproval. The individual worker is expected to put his or her *Uchi* group before self-interest (Hendry 1995).

Activity 13.1

In what ways do you think work in modern capitalist societies differs from work in pre-industrial societies? You might like to think about the structure of the working day or year and whether work is carried out by individuals or groups.

WORK TODAY AND THE DIVISION OF LABOUR

Work in modern societies consists of thousands of different tasks and occupations. The sheer diversity of modern work contrasts with simpler and smaller-scale modes of work practised in earlier hunter-gatherer or feudal societies. In previous forms of society, people would engage in one single task, seeing it through from onset to completion. For example, a carpenter would oversee the production of a chair from the moment he cut and prepared the wood to the moment the varnish dried and the completed chair was sold to a customer. Today, many people would be employed in the same task of producing a chair, each being responsible for one small part of the overall process, such as turning the legs on a lathe or spraying the varnish onto the constituent components. Each worker labours without knowledge of the others and without any say in the end product.

It was the development of capitalism and the Industrial Revolution that generated the vast array of types of work we know today. An important concept that describes this style of work in modern society is that of 'division of labour'. While this form of social organization reaches its height in capitalist societies, all societies possess some form of division of labour. In pre-industrial societies, this may take the form of elementary distinctions between the work that men or women do, or between those involved in crafts or agriculture. Historically, as has been mentioned, one worker was responsible for one all-encompassing craft task, but in modern societies, we find thousands and thousands of tasks and jobs in which people are engaged. This is known as the division of labour, whereby different people specialize in distinct and discrete tasks. The previous example of the many different people involved in manufacturing a chair illustrates how labour is divided in modern-day industrial production.

Other examples of the division of labour are evident throughout society. For example, when it comes to the sexual division of labour, there exists a wealth of sex-differentiated tasks in both paid employment and other activities that someone could potentially be paid to do (Oakley 1985a). Men are still, even after successive campaigns and legislation to bring about greater equality, more likely to engage in DIY or car maintenance, leaving women to take care of food preparation and the dishes afterwards (Jowell et al 1992). Inside health care, there are also a number of examples of the division of labour.

Medical workers are divided into a number of specialized areas: surgeons, doctors, physiotherapists, occupational therapists, etc. Within those broad divisions, there will exist further divisions of labour and specializations, for example therapists who specialize in psychiatric or physical rehabilitation.

Activity 13.2

Can you identify some more examples of the division of labour, either within or outside health care?

HOW DOES WORK AFFECT OUR LIVES?

In addition to the wider aspects of work in society, work affects our lives in more immediate and concrete ways. The following four functions of work are identified by Victor (1994) as being universal to the experience of paid work:

- income
- structure
- social status
- social relationships.

Income

This is fairly obvious. Basically, in a modern capitalist society, it is very difficult to have any standard of living without an income. It is with money that we purchase the necessities to live and the other goods and activities that make life worth living.

Structure

Since we spend a large percentage of our time working, it becomes an important organizing principle in our lives. In Britain and other countries, the average working week is increasing to somewhere around 40 hours. It is around the portion of the day devoted to working that other activities such as leisure, family and other social relationships are based. You may have experienced for yourself how initially disorientating it can be when you have an extended break from work. You may have found it difficult to get out of bed in the morning without a specific purpose.

Social status

In addition to income and structure, work provides a certain amount of social status, often reflected in the wage that is paid. Higher-status jobs generally have higher wages, at least in the long run. So for example, in many countries, doctors who may have a high status start their careers on a relatively low salary compared with some of their graduate friends, but their long-term earning potential is greater.

Social relationships

The other three functions are all vital to our experience of work, but for many people it is how well we get on with our fellow workers that is important. Considering how much time is invested in work, it is a common place for new and old social relationships to be organized.

Activity 13.3

Make a list of those things about work which are important to you. Compare your list with those of your colleagues.

THEORIES OF WORK

As with other areas of sociology, it is simply not enough to describe a particular event; it is also necessary to attempt to understand why people behave in certain ways. This is where theory comes in. Theories relating to work offer a viewpoint that may cut against some 'common-sense' interpretations of work, for example that people do not work hard because they are lazy. Marx would contend that people may not 'work hard' because they have little control over their work, which is boring or routine, and as a consequence feel apathetic towards it.

Marx and work

Marx contributed greatly to our theoretical understanding of work within modern capitalist society. The majority of his work focused on analysing the vast changes in society that were happening at the time of the Industrial Revolution. He attempted to provide an understanding of the emergence of capitalism as an industrial and social force that was transforming every aspect of life, from individual relationships to the organization of the nation state. In examining the shift towards an industrial mode of production (work being carried out in factories with a high division of labour, etc.), Marx wrote extensively about the organization and role of work. Indeed, for Marx, work was, as we saw in Chapter 2, an essential aspect of being human.

In many ways, Marx's ideas on the centrality of work to our existence are similar to occupational therapy's perspectives on the human need for occupation (Wilcock 1993). For Marx, it is our capacity for work that produces society, culture and social interaction. By our collective labour, we act upon the natural and physical world around us, and by changing that world, we alter and transform the social world as well. As Marx (1867) notes, 'by thus acting on the external world and changing it, he [sic] at the same time changes his own nature'.

What Marx is basically observing is that, without work, we as humans, both individually and socially, could not advance. The processes of work are the building blocks of what makes humanity unique. Animals merely react to the outside world, while we, as active beings with intelligence and creativity, act upon the world and shape it for our needs. When we quarry stone to build shelter, we not only keep the rain off, but also create spaces that hold important social interactions. An assembly of stones can be a house or a church, each denoting a host of different relationships and statements about a particular society. Without work, we would be denying what Marx terms 'our species nature'.

This may give the impression that Marx was an avid supporter of work, perhaps viewing it as a pleasurable experience in which people willingly engage. However, for many people, work is an activity that is, if not hated, then disliked. We would all rather be doing something other than working. Marx also realized this and observed that work under modern-day capitalism is a repetitive and boring task: that is to say, it is alienating.

Alienation

The reason Marx puts forward to explain this is that work under modern capitalism alienates the worker from his or her work. This concept of alienation identifies that workers have little or no control over the work itself and that the work is more powerful and important than the individual worker. This powerlessness comes about as a result of the division of labour today, being fragmented into so many constituent parts that the worker has no control over the overall process. This results in the alienated worker feeling a sense of powerlessness, isolation and indifference towards her work. The only reason that she carries on working is that, in a capitalist society, she will not be able to survive without the income that working provides. Marx identified four types of alienation (adapted from Slattery 1990):

• Loss of control of the end product. The worker has no say in what happens to what she has produced. Instead, it is the employer who takes control

• Loss of involvement in production process. Here the worker regards him or herself as a mere component within the whole production process, the only incentive to work being the wage at the end of the day

• Rivalling others: Under capitalism, workers are often pitted against each other for bonuses and promotion, while the employer exerts unequal power over the workforce

• Denial of self expression: The work is no longer an intrinsic part of the worker and does not reflect her skills and abilities

The common theme running throughout the above is one of the worker being subsumed by the process of work, all aspects of the worker's control, individuality and creativity being marginalized.

Weber and work

Weber, like Marx, also analysed the structures of society, searching for unifying themes that could explain the great changes brought about by the advance of capitalism and the Industrial Revolution. In many ways, Weber has an outlook similar to that of Marx, but he differs in some fundamental ways. Weber sought to identify social action and ideal types as an approach to understanding the modern state and was interested in how ideas affect and influence changes in society. This is a different approach from that of Marx, who relied mainly on examining the economic relationships between different classes. A key part of Weber's overall analysis is the effect that the Protestant ethic (more commonly known as the work ethic) had in shaping modern capitalism.

Weber noted the similarity between the values of capitalism and the values of Protestantism. Both place a reliance on hard work, individualism, rational organization and, most importantly, the pursuit of profit. Of particular importance was the element of austerity within Protestantism. Thus, although profit was something good, to spend it on fancy goods and show was not. This therefore left the way open for the re-investment of profit into business, which in turn created more profit. Weber claimed that, as part of the overall change to capitalism, the influence of the Protestant ethic was important in forming pro-work attitudes and beliefs. With people believing in the Protestant ethic, the progress of capitalism and the modern-day concept of working were made possible. These attitudes and beliefs are visible around us today. Many people feel an important commitment to work, and great emphasis is placed on working hard and well. The consequences of the work ethic will be discussed further in the next section.

UNEMPLOYMENT

Long-term unemployment is now endemic within many sectors of the global economy. As a result of the 1973 oil crisis, successive downturns in the economy and the expansion of automated

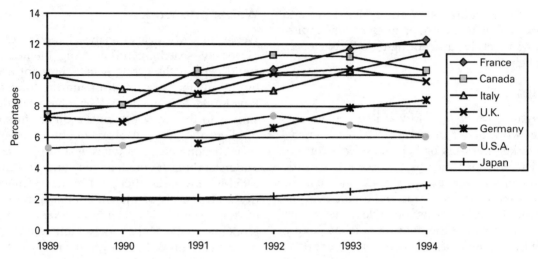

Figure 13.1 Unemployment rates adjusted to SOEC* concepts: G7 comparison (CSO 1996).
*Except Canada, which is based on OECD concepts

assembly techniques, the accepted belief in a 'job for life' can now be severely questioned. As the statistics above (Fig. 13.1) indicate, unemployment in two of the most advanced industrial countries – Britain and the USA – has risen steadily over the past few decades. Indeed, unemployment is a common experience for all of the G7 economic countries. Caution must, however, be urged when consulting official government statistics. This is because definitions of unemployment have changed with successive administrations and because the extent of unemployment may be, in some ways, 'hidden'.

Unemployment is not entirely random, certain social groups being more vulnerable to it than others. Those belonging to ethnic groups, young people and working-class people are generally much more likely to be unemployed or be threatened with unemployment.

The physical, psychological and social effects of unemployment are well documented (Crick 1981, Fineman 1987, Kelvin & Jarrett 1985, Oppenheim & Harker 1996). Basically, unemployment sees the negation of the four functions of work listed below.

Income

The loss of income is a major crisis for many unemployed people. The Child Poverty Action Group (CPAG) noted that, in Britain, unemployment benefit was 13.8% of average income. This led to unemployed families cutting back expenditure on food, clothing and entertainment, their disposable income being 59% of what it was prior to unemployment (Oppenheim & Harker 1996).

Structure

Even if a job is extremely dull and tedious, it still provides some organizational structure. The sudden emptiness created by unemployment can lead to depression and apathy, the unemployed person finding difficulty in engaging in new activities to replace ones lost as a result of becoming unemployed.

Social status

The strong relationship between work and social status influences how people feel about themselves when unemployed. The identity and self-esteem that they once would have found in their work is gone. This is especially relevant to men, who depend largely on their work for feelings of self-worth.

Social interaction

Without the familiar routines and patterns of work, the unemployed person may find it difficult to maintain relationships that they had in the workplace and consequently to make new ones. The attachment to the work ethic is an important influence in coping with unemployment. Research has found that the more closely someone identifies with the work ethic, the more problems he or she has in dealing with unemployment. For many, there is a strong sense of stigma associated with not being in work. Douthwaite (1994) suggests that occupational therapists should assist unemployed people by helping them reduce their commitment to work and devising strategies that will encourage positive use of the increases in time created by unemployment.

Activity 13.4

Have you, or has someone you know, experienced an extended period of unemployment? What effects did it have?

WOMEN AND WORK

As with other areas of sociology, as highlighted in Chapter 6, there has in the past tended to be a male bias in the study of work. This is apparent in sociological analyses of work stressing male-oriented paid work. Pahl (1984), after research on informal work practices on the Isle of Sheppey, noted that 'This neglect may be explained partially by the emphasis on the individual wage earner, rather than the household, as the basic economic unit.'

A focus on male aspects of work can lead to diminishing the work of women and the particular differences of women's work and the sexual division of labour. This often leads to the depiction that men work and women do not – hence the saying '*just* a housewife'. Research and the influence of feminist sociology highlight a different picture, as McDonnell & Pringle (1992) comment about work and women: 'they have not been excluded from work but they have too much work'.

The double burden

In discussing work, it is vital not to ignore the role that domestic labour plays in the lives of women. Women, especially working-class women, face the 'double burden' of having to work for a wage in addition to carrying out domestic labour. The optimism of early researchers, such as Young & Willmott (1973), or the rise of the 'new man', suggested that an equal division of household labour was on its way. Unfortunately, statistical and research evidence indicates that that household tasks still tend to be gender biased.

As Figure 13.2 illustrates, there are a number

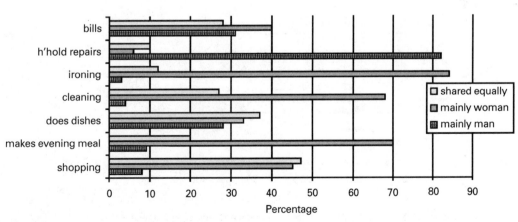

Figure 13.2 Who performs household tasks? (Data from Jowell et al, 1992.)

of household tasks that display a certain degree of inequality. Household repairs, a stereotypical male activity, are still quite male centred, while the household chores of cleaning and ironing are still the responsibility of women. Oakley's (1976, 1985b) classic studies of housework revealed the similarities between domestic and non-domestic labour. Both forms of work can be characterized by an endless routine of repetitive and unfulfilling tasks. Many women also commented on the 'invisible' nature and low status of housework, which added to the lack of recognition that domestic labour receives. Some women, however, did report that they enjoyed the control that they had in planning and organizing various household tasks.

When examining paid labour outside the home, a number of other inequalities are apparent, in terms of earnings, types of work and full- and part-time work. A woman will typically have a low earning, part-time job that is likely to be in the service sector or the 'caring professions'. Even though there have been many legislative attempts to reduce the disparity in wage earning, there still exists a gulf between the incomes of men and women. Figure 13.3 illustrates the differences in earning power.

A similar disparity exists in the USA. The median earnings for a male accountant in 1989 were $34 867, while a female accountant could expect $22 960. A male computer operator's median earnings were $23 066, whereas his female counterpart would receive $16 849 (US Bureau of the Census 1989, cited in Brinkerhoff et al 1992). There are a number of reasons for this:

- Women are more likely to work in smaller companies
- Women are more likely to work part time
- A woman's employment flexibility and promotional opportunities will be affected by children and family responsibilities. The lack of adequate childcare facilities will limit where a woman can choose to live and work as well as the times she can work
- Outright discrimination is another factor – women have to contend with the 'glass ceiling' effect, whereby they can see the top jobs but are prevented from reaching them by discriminatory or sexist attitudes held by male employers
- The types of work available to women, discussed further below.

Women's work

Men and women tend to work in quite different areas. In Britain, approximately one-quarter of employed men as opposed to one in 10 employed women, work in manufacturing. However, when it comes to health, there are four times as many women as men. Women are also overrepresented in clerical and secretarial jobs, a quarter of employed women working in those areas (Central

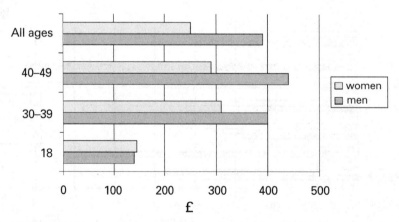

Figure 13.3 Income differences between men and women in Britain at selected ages (*from CSO 1996*).

Statistical Office 1996). Again, there exist similar patterns in the USA. Forty-five per cent of employed women work in sales and clerical, as opposed to 20% of men, while precision production accounts for 21% of employed men compared with 2% of women (US Department of Labour 1990, cited in Brinkerhoff et al 1992).

Activity 13.5

Why is it that some jobs are considered to be 'women's work'? Chapter 6 will give you some answers.

From what you have read so far, you will have gained an appreciation that work is a complex concept with different meanings for different individuals in different contexts. In addition, the nature of work appears to be changing over time, especially since the decline of the Industrial Revolution in the Western world and the development of what has been called postindustrialism. We now need to consider how this relates to occupational therapy.

WORK AND OCCUPATIONAL THERAPY

As occupational therapists, we have a long history of using work and work-related activity as therapy. Work as therapy aims to impart skills, facilitate mastery of the environment, improve self-esteem and confidence through social interaction and offer individuals more control over their lives (Harvey-Krefting 1985). The therapeutic use of work has always been viewed as positive, but we may have to change our firmly held beliefs since not everybody has or will have secure paid employment in the future. So how should we use this information to shape our thoughts about work and our intervention?

This part of this chapter will explore the following issues:

- What is the relationship between work and human occupation within the profession of occupational therapy?

- How should occupational therapists view work within their practice?
- Should occupational therapists assist the able bodied and people with disabilities to gain work and deal with the effects of unemployment?

Activity 13.6

Discuss what work means to you personally.

HUMAN OCCUPATION

The question in Activity 13.6 would probably produce different responses from different people since no universal agreement exists at this time about definitions of work. This is particularly true within occupational therapy, and our understanding of these themes is continually evolving and changing. However, as pointed out in the previous part of this chapter, most people in the Western world tend to associate work with status and pay in order to maintain their 'lifestyle', although this appears to be changing. This change is due to the advancement of technology and the reduction in the number of full-time jobs available throughout a person's working life (Farnworth 1995).

As occupational therapists, the philosophical and humanistic base of our profession tends to construct our particular view of work (and especially paid work) in a certain manner, i.e. work is only *one* aspect of human occupation. In other words, occupational therapists perceive human occupation as being much broader than just the singular issue of work, whether paid or not. The developing discipline of occupational science attempts to address this issue.

Occupational science

Some individuals in our profession, such as Wilcock (1993), would state that human occupation is 'the purposeful use of time, energy, interest and attention in work, self-care and leisure activities'. The emerging discipline of occupational science attempts to clarify the relationship between

---

Box 13.1 Occupational science (Wilcock 1993)

Occupational science is the rigorous study of:

- the human need to be occupied
- the purpose of occupation in survival and health
- the effects of occupation or occupation deprivation
- why humans strive for occupational competence and mastery
- understanding what prevents or enhances occupational performance
- how social, cultural and political structures affect occupation
- how occupation provides for biological and sociocultural needs
- how occupation is necessary in the development of human capacities

---

human occupation and the importance of work, self-care and leisure. The definition of the scope of occupational science can be seen in Box 13.1.

As stated in the previous part of this chapter, some of the themes above are similar to Marx's view that working is a central part of being human. As occupational therapists, we need to reflect on the importance of sociological theories about work and how this 'articulates' with our broader interpretation and view of human occupation, which also values the importance of self-care and leisure.

Within the context of human occupation, what 'self-care' and 'leisure' activities constitute is probably to some degree self-explanatory, but how is work currently defined in the minds of occupational therapists?

The conceptualization of work in occupational therapy

Occupational therapists, especially in America and Canada (Jacobs 1991, Kielhofner 1985, Law et al 1990), believe that a wide range of human activities can be classified as work.

Occupational therapists utilizing models of practice centred on human occupation believe that work is applicable throughout the whole of the lifespan rather than just in adulthood, so young children, teenagers, adults and the elderly can also therefore be engaged in work. Additionally, another important factor is that occupational therapists do not necessarily equate work

solely with financial reward, and therefore other areas, including voluntary work and working in retirement, are very important in terms of life satisfaction.

Using the statements above as a basis for what could be classified as 'work', Jacobs (1991) describes the following:

1. *Home management*: This includes buying and caring for clothes, cleaning the house, planning and preparing meals, shopping, managing money, and maintenance and safety considerations in and around the house

2. *Care of others*: This infers providing for and supporting children, looking after spouses' and parents' needs, attending to others' physical care, communicating and determining others' needs and carrying out these activities in a manner that is appropriate to the age of the person

3. *Educational activities*: This involves attending nursery, primary and secondary school and/or a college or university environment, doing homework, assignments, exams, etc., studying, seeking further training, retraining and being involved in extracurricular activities with others

4. *Vocational activities (paid or voluntary)*: Thinking about different types of work, ways of finding out about different types of work, contacting employers and agencies, filling in application forms, attending interviews, maintaining worker performance and, importantly, retirement planning.

Activity 13.7

Which of the above activities would you consider as work, and why? Would you describe any of them as leisure?

Classifying and categorizing definitions (as above) helps us to focus our thoughts more clearly on a complex issue, but according to some people, not all of the activities above might be thought of as work. As occupational therapists, we have to keep an open mind about individuals' interpretations of what constitutes work and be aware of gender, culture and class issues. This broad interpretation of work is consistent with the philosophy of occupational therapy that views human beings in a 'biopsychosocial perspective' (Hubbard 1991), that is, recognizing humans as biological beings with feelings, emotions, opinions and needs that change over time; who interact with and are shaped by each other and their environment. It is important for occupational therapists to act in a way that reflects this broad view of human occupation, especially when intervening in a therapeutic manner in relation to managing work issues with clients. In other words, what people think about work, their lives and what shapes their opinions is important, and occupational therapists ought to respect their position.

THE PLACE OF WORK IN PEOPLE'S LIVES

As mentioned earlier in this chapter, work (in the context of human occupation) is an important aspect of our lives and may in many ways affects 'who we are'. From a sociological perspective, work may structure and organize our time (past, present and future) and therefore provide meaning in our lives. Personal roles, status and identity, and establishing and maintaining social roles, are also important aspects of work. Work also fulfils need in society: it may act as a means for social interaction, personal and shared achievement, it can signal recovery from illness, and it may provide financial reward (Holmes 1985). However, as we have already seen, there are negative aspects to work.

There are disadvantages associated with being in work in terms of alienation (as defined by Marx). This is reflected in not feeling in control of one's future, being in active competition with other colleagues or other larger businesses and not feeling valued or rewarded by employers. Of course, if work is central to human experience and deemed to be important in society, people who are out of work face a different set of problems. These problems may include being stigmatized in terms of being seen as 'lazy' (consider the Protestant ethic mentioned earlier in this chapter), loss of status and role, poverty and the associated loss of social interaction, which can

collectively lead to long-term mental health and physical problems.

Work and health

Many people experience overwork, which appears to be evident in terms of the increasing number of hours people spend working, and may also experience a range of problems. For example, stress, both physical and psychological, according to Pratt (1996), costs British industry 90 million lost working days in terms of absenteeism, at an annual cost of £7 billion. Other problems include 'burn out', fear of the future regarding financial security, physical consequences (ulcers, heart disease), boredom (Armstrong & McKay 1996), sustaining acute injuries (impairment), chronic injury (disability) and long-term pain. For example, chronic pain can be a consequence of repetitive strain injury (RSI), which, according to some (Chalmers 1993, Fast 1995), is reaching epidemic proportions in the workplace as costs are reduced and more work is expected in terms of efficiency gains. Although more productive work is encouraged by employers, its detrimental side-effects and long-term consequences may still be viewed by the employer as 'laziness' and 'malingering behaviour'.

People who are disabled and have work or are unemployed experience additional problems, for example being dependent on carers and the benefits system, encountering discrimination in the workplace, possibly having to take extended periods of sick leave and having to overcome architectural barriers at work such as stairs and heavy doors.

OCCUPATIONAL THERAPY INTERVENTION AND WORK

Occupational therapists do or can intervene and manage work-related issues at several different levels and in different locations. Consider how occupational therapists could be of assistance to people who are:

- in danger of sustaining physical injury through repetitive tasks at work

- temporarily out of work because of acute injury
- experiencing chronic pain because of repetitive injuries while working
- unemployed in the long term
- disabled and wishing to find work
- disabled and experiencing problems coping with the requirements and demands of their work.

Occupational therapists can offer help to employers and employees in the workplace in terms of advice and education programmes, environmental adaptations, health promotion programmes, ergonomic advice and intervention to help people prevent RSI and stress in the workplace (Armstrong & McKay 1996). For example by assessing whether a person is using the computer keyboard efficiently while seated at the desk in order to maximize comfort and prevent injury.

Occupational therapists may also be part of a pain management programme that helps people to re-educate themselves about managing their pain, its effects on their relationships and how to pace themselves physically to avoid exacerbating their condition. This programme would also help the individual to set new goals, for example in relation to finding employment, ultimately promoting more control, independence and self-esteem.

Occupational therapy and unemployment

Occupational therapists help people who are temporarily unemployed through injury. This involves an attempt to remedy workers' problems by assessing their work skills and being involved in therapeutic programmes in order for them to secure competitive employment. This has been the case, for example, in America, where work rehabilitation centres are evident. These multidisciplinary centres assist people by assessing the capacity for work, offering retraining, work-hardening programmes, education about injuries and skill development, thereby helping the injured person back to work. Supported employment schemes have also been developed to assist those previously considered unemployable (for example, people with severe learning disbilities) to get into work. An example of this type of work is given in Chapter 15.

Dealing with the short-term effects of unemployment by utilizing other meaningful activities and leisure, helping people come to terms with unemployment and issues related to securing future employment may also be useful. Consequently, occupational therapists need to be aware of current legislation regarding opportunities for training schemes, etc, and also to liaise with appropriate government and training and support agencies that assist people to participate in paid employment. For example, in Britain, Disability Employment Advisors within the Placing, Assessment and Counselling Teams (PACT) are located at the Employment Agency.

> **Activity 13.8**
>
> Find out what schemes exist in your area to help disabled people or people with mental health problems to gain employment.

In relation to unemployment, Douthwaite, an occupational therapist (1994), enquires whether occupational therapists should *only* concern themselves with the consequences of long-term unemployment, that is when people in their practice become ill apparently from not having work (e.g. suffering from depression, anxiety or physical impairment. She considers that occupational therapists ought to offer assistance in relation to helping people to combat the negative effects of loss of role through unemployment by providing opportunities to examine the significance of work and leisure in their lives and the psychological consequences of employment and unemployment, learning to cope through group work and helping to develop future plans. In other words, occupational therapists may have to realize that 'getting a job' should not necessarily dominate every aspect of a person's life and that some individuals may be 'at a higher risk of breakdown physically or psychologically' if they return to work (Steward 1996).

Similarly, Primeau (1996) believes that occupational therapists attempting to restore healthy, balanced lifestyles as a priority, by reinforcing a traditional belief in equal amounts of work, rest and play as positive, does not help some people and may have a tendency to reinforce the 'Protestant work ethic'. Occupational therapists need to study the sociological aspects of work within the context of human occupation and understand what 'health' means to particular individuals. Finally, seeing beyond common-sense beliefs held by society in terms of finding employment at all costs or consequently being labelled as 'lazy' may have to be revisited as more people find themselves unemployed.

CONCLUSION

Hopefully, by now, work can be seen as a much more complex and multidimensional phenomenon than simply turning up at the workplace at 9 in the morning and disappearing at 5. To offer a simple definition of work is, in many cases, as pointless as it is difficult, owing to the vast variety of tasks and occupations that constitute the activities of all human beings. This is not to say that various sociological theories, such as those of Marx and Weber, cannot illuminate the reasons why particular forms of work exist or help us to understand the importance of work within our lives.

You have read that work is a complex concept and that no definite answers are readily available for solving these issues. Occupational therapists need to turn their attention to examining what human occupation, self-care, work and leisure mean for people in their own lives. Additionally, occupational therapists can be involved in managing people who do have work-related problems. Through our undergraduate education, we are well placed to understand the psychosocial and physical implications of injury impeding work, undertaking assessment and post-programme evaluation, using therapeutic media that are meaningful to improve skills and endurance, and modifying attitudes and architectural barriers through practice grounded in occupational therapy models, treatment approaches and educational and ergonomic principles.

REFERENCES

Armstrong J, McKay M 1996 Occupational stress: an interactionist perspective. British Journal of Therapy and Rehabilitation 3(1): 25–29
Brinkerhoff D, White L, Ortega S 1992 Essentials of sociology. West, St Paul, MN
Chalmers F 1993 The non-existent disease of epidemic proportions. Therapy Weekly, 18 Nov: 4
Crick B (ed.) 1981 Unemployment. Methuen, London
CSO 1996 Social trends. HMSO, London
Douthwaite J 1994 Unemployment: a challenge to occupational therapy. British Journal of Occupational Therapy 57(11): 432–436
Farnworth L 1995 An exploration of skill as an issue in employment and unemployment. Australian Journal of Occupational Science 2(1): 22–29
Fast C 1995 Repetitive strain injury: an overview of the condition and its implications for occupational therapy. Canadian Journal of Occupational Therapy 62(3): 119–126
Fineman S 1987 Unemployment: personal and social consequences. Tavistock, London
Grint K 1991 The sociology of work. Blackwell, Oxford
Harvey-Krefting L 1985 The concept of work in occupational therapy: a historical review. American Journal of Occupational Therapy 39(5): 301–307
Hendry J 1995 Understanding Japanese society, 2nd edn.

Routledge, London
Holmes D 1985 The role of the occupational therapist – work evaluator. American Journal of Occupational Therapy 39(5): 308–313
Hubbard S 1991 Towards a truly holistic approach to occupational therapy. British Journal of Occupational Therapy 54(11): 415–418
Jacobs K 1991 Occupational therapy: work related programmes and assessment. Little, Brown, Boston
Jowell R et al (eds) 1992 British social attitudes: the 9th report. Dartmouth, Aldershot
Kelvin P, Jarrett J 1985 Unemployment: its social psychological effects. European Monograph in Social Psychology
Kielhofner G 1985 A model of human occupation. Williams & Wilkins; Baltimore
Law M, Baptiste S, McColl M A, Opzoomer A, Polatajko H, Pollock N 1990 The Canadian Occupational Performance Measure: an outcome measure for occupational therapy. Canadian Journal of Occupational Therapy 57(2): 82–87
McDonnell, Pringle 1992 Defining women. OUP, London
Marx K 1867 Capital 1. In Wilcock A 1993 A theory of human need. Journal of Occupational Science 1(1)
Oakley A 1976 Housewife. Penguin, Harmondsworth
Oakley A 1985a Sex, gender and society. Gower Maurice Temple Smith, Hampshire

Oakley A 1985b The sociology of housework. Blackwell, Oxford

Oppenheim C, Harker L 1996 Poverty: the facts, 3rd edn. Child Poverty Action Group, London

Pahl R 1984 Divisions of labour. Blackwell, Oxford

Pratt J 1996 Taking occupational therapy into the workplace. British Journal of Therapy and Rehabilitation 3(1): 21–24

Primeau L 1996 Work and Leisure: rethinking leisure theory Sage, London

Sahlins M 1972 Stone Age Economics Aldine, Chicago

Slattery M 1990 Key ideas in sociology. Macmillan, Basingstoke

Steward B 1996 Unemployment and Health, 2: The implications of unemployment for therapy and rehabilitation. British Journal of Therapy and Rehabilitation 3(8): 426–447

Victor C 1994 Old age in modern society: a textbook of social gerontology. Chapman & Hall, London

Wilcock A A 1993 Editorial. Journal of Occupational Science 1(1): 1–2

Young M, Willmott P 1973 The symmetrical family: a study of work and leisure in the London regien. Routledge & Kegan Paul, London

14

Leisure

Louise R. Thibodaux

Anita C. Bundy

THE COMPLEX NATURE OF LEISURE

Leisure is obviously of prime concern to occupational therapists, and later in this chapter we will look at some specific issues for therapists. However, one may ask why the study of leisure should be of concern in the social sciences. Dumazedier, a key sociologist in this field of study, provides a straightforward answer to this question by observing that leisure 'has a deep-going intricate interrelatedness to the largest questions of work, family and politics' (1967, p. 4). This interrelatedness is viewed from a variety of perspectives even by social scientists themselves. Economists might answer that leisure is important because developed countries such as the USA spend up to 7% of family income on leisure activities (Kelly & Godbey 1992). Sociologists might observe that activities which are identified as leisure often occur in groups or affect the interactions of people and groups. Group behaviour, sociologists have pointed out, is normative behaviour. Compare, for example, the way in which one acts at a garden party to one's behaviour at a football match. Anthropologists might focus on the symbolic meaning inherent in leisure transactions. An employer may 'give' a day off work, but the hobbyist 'takes' pleasure in flowers from the garden or in a product from the sewing room (Kelly 1983).

All would agree that leisure as 'free time' provides opportunities for personal as well as group expression (Cutler & Hendricks 1990). In fact, 'freedom' and 'time' are central leisure concepts.

As is true of all other freedoms, free time has personal, cultural, economic and political consequences (Dumazedier 1967). In many ways, the leisure choices made by individuals serve as mirrors, reflecting the influences of ideology, technology and demography within each society (Kelly & Godbey 1992).

Although leisure activity is central to the human experience, leisure can mean different things to different people. To a farmer, leisure may mean time to look at next year's seed catalogues; to a businessman, leisure may mean a week in Florida or the South of France; to a computer operator, leisure may mean the chance to play a game of tennis. Nelson (1988) suggests that the meaning attributed to any activity is embedded within the form that the activity takes. If he is correct, there is also an explicit link between the need to experience meaning through leisure and the forms, both individual and collective, of leisure occupations.

DEFINING LEISURE

Joffre Dumazedier (1967, pp. 16–17) offers a definition of leisure that is broad enough to encompass a wide variety of forms and meanings:

Leisure is activity – apart from the obligations of work, family, and society – to which the individual turns at will for either relaxation, diversion, or broadening of his knowledge and his spontaneous social participation, the free exercise of his creative capacity.

This definition points out that leisure is distinct from work and also from other activities that may not be freely chosen by the individual. The focus in leisure may be on relaxation, diversion or social participation. Furthermore, the way in which one experiences leisure may be influenced by one's current life circumstances as well as one's past interests and the interests of one's own

social circle (Neulinger 1981). The central feature of leisure, distinguishing it from other types of human activity, is that the meaning of the act itself is freely determined by the person who performs it.

Imagine the fly-fisherman wading into a stream. He may find that the activity offers compensatory relaxation because it helps to diffuse the stresses and strains of modern life; it may be habitual when it is part of a weekend pattern or when it is experienced by returning to the same place over and over again; or it may be social because it represents a commitment to status or to a specific way of life. Recreational fishing is a good example of a single activity that fulfils all these functions simultaneously.

The key dimensions of leisure that have been of most interest to social scientists centre around how participation is affected by time, the cultural meaning of the activity and the interior attitude of the participant (Box 14.1).

Despite the neatness of this chart, the exact features that constitute leisure have been termed a 'conceptual morass' (Cutler & Hendricks 1990, p. 169). Perhaps it is for this reason that, of occupational forms within modern life, the study of leisure has received the least attention. Research into leisure has used a mixture of concepts and methods, making theory-building difficult for sociologists.

Activity 14.1

Make a list of all the things you enjoy as leisure activities. How are these different from work activities? Do you experience different degrees of pleasure from different activities?
    Compare your list with that of one of your colleagues.

Box 14.1   Facets of leisure

Leisure is:

A kind of time	Free from obligation Non-essential activity Performed in spare time Time without pressure Lasts temporarily Self-rewarding
Culturally defined activity	Bounded by social norms Provides individual status Varies according to groups Changes across the lifespan Organized in patterns
Interior attitude	Pleasurable, relaxing Exploratory Freely chosen Liberating Intrinsically motivated

CONCEPTUAL AND METHODOLOGICAL QUAGMIRES

The sociological concepts used to define leisure incorporate both subjective and objective dimensions (Neulinger 1981). Even when there appears to be some agreement regarding some elements of leisure, conceptual and methodological difficulties have blocked the development of a unified approach to its study. Problems include the following:

- the element of free choice
- the tendency to identify leisure with left-over time, in comparison with 'serious work' time
- the nature of individual meaning
- the spontaneous nature of leisure expression.

Leisure as free choice

People choose leisure freely. This means that they are in control from moment to moment of the type of activity, the pace of the activity and the purpose of activity. A bystander watching an activity has few clues about how engagement is 'fine-tuned' by a succession of choices. In that sense, leisure participation becomes a creative activity that appears to take on a life of its own.

Activity 14.2

1. Think about the last time you did something that lasted over 20 minutes 'for fun'. Can you remember changing your pace, changing your level of interest? When did you know it was time to stop?

2. If you are a person who has little time for leisure or who feels guilty about 'wasting time', consider the reasons. What is stopping you from 'joyfully affirming your place in the universe'?

Leisure as time use

It is tempting to think of leisure solely as un-obligated time when a person can 'kick back' and do something just for fun. Actually, it is much more complicated than that. Shopping is a good example of an activity that combines elements of work and leisure. Some people are 'power shoppers', while others are 'mall loungers'. It might be hard for the observer to distinguish which is work and which is play.

Activity 14.3

Do you do anything in your leisure time that other people might think of as work? Do you do anything at work that others might view as leisure?

Leisure and individual meaning

Human beings are meaning-seekers and meaning-makers. Although animals have been observed to frolic, none except humans seems to rely on leisure as a primary way of relating to the world. People who are depressed and cannot enjoy life often describe a profound loss of the ability to be spontaneous (Karp 1996). Leisure connects us with the symbolic energy that is the wellspring of life and health.

Activity 14.4

Without using words, draw how you feel when you are engaged in leisure. Show the drawing to a colleague and tell him or her why it is important to you.

Leisure as spontaneous expression

Imagine trying to study an event that was so spontaneous that you never knew quite when it was going to happen. This is one of the problems with studying leisure. The mind-set of leisure is 'fun-loving' and 'carefree'. People cannot tell you: 'Watch me, I think I'm about to have fun.' The best way to study leisure is to ask people to talk about things that they enjoy. Even then, it is difficult to know why they consider one activity leisure and another work. It is also difficult to know exactly how much time anyone actually spends in leisure since data are gathered from personal recollections. For this reason, social scientists have often used financial expenditure as a proxy measurement.

As a starting point, then, let us agree with Dumazedier (1967) that, when pursuing leisure, one is entirely free to exercise one's full autonomy and creative potential. By adopting this inclusive definition, we affirm that all have 'abilities' for leisure even when physical or mental impairments might hamper participation in particular types of activity or modify the way in which they are performed.

CLASSICAL PERSPECTIVES

Classical theories in sociology have described leisure from a variety of perspectives. The perspectives of functionalism, conflict theory and symbolic interaction summarized in Box 14.2 are discussed at length below.

Box 14.2   Traditional sociological perspectives

Functionalism	Meets need for social survival
	Creation of cohesive social bonds
	Promotes defined social roles
	Reinforces normative responses
	Creates community feeling
	May involve participation in ritual
Conflict theory	Based on competition for resources
	Expresses power relationships
	Involves winners and losers
Symbolic interaction	Participation creates meaning
	Open expression and self-development
	Use of instruments, forms and symbols
	A temporary psychosocial state
	Links time, attitude and experience

Functionalism

The focus of functionalism is on the social cohesion produced by particular human activities. According to this perspective, forms of leisure meet the need to contribute to social survival because they support productivity and social bonding (Jarvie & Maguire 1994). Participation in specific activities, for example choral music or athletic contests, builds self-discipline and teaches the skills necessary for teamwork. Group participation in leisure serves both to form and to define the common interests necessary for civic and national pride. Leisure maintains social bonds because it provides the time and social space both for the development of the self and for the development of intimate relationships with others.

This generally positive view of leisure was not, however, espoused by early sociologists. Emile Durkheim wrote that 'the need to play, to indulge in acting without any purpose and for the pleasure of so doing cannot be developed beyond a certain point without detaching oneself from the serious business of life' (Durkheim 1893 [1984], p. 185). Veblen (1899 [1965]) expressed a similar suspicion about leisure, which he criticized for being time-consuming without giving back any visible product to society. Underlying these criticisms is the belief that a hedonistically playful orientation toward life can have negative consequences for society as a whole. Although early theorists saw leisure's contribution to societal cohesion as 'either/or', recent theorists have pointed out that it is more a case of 'both/and' (Caillois 1979). Nevertheless, there will always be an embedded tension between the 'serious' and the 'non-serious' as far as leisure is concerned. This unresolved tension reinforces the view that leisure and work are separate.

Activity 14.5: Functional perspective

Which of your leisure activities links you to a larger social unit? What kinds of event do you celebrate: family events, community events, national holidays? Would you describe these activities as more 'serious' or more 'non-serious'?

Conflict theory

The major contribution of conflict theory is its perspective on the interplay of power relationships between different segments of society. Several types of leisure pursuit, specifically sport and contests of various kinds, externalize the struggle for power (Luschen & Sage 1981). Leisure itself can be considered to be a mirror of social values because the form and purpose of public activities often represent underlying social attitudes. For example, Western capitalist societies whose economy is based on values of competition, achievement and prowess provide for winning and losing through organized sports. While contestants on the field compete with each other, their fans, dressed in the colours of the team, cheer from the sidelines. Drinking after the game reinforces the fact that participants and fans are 'part of the team'. Small wonder that women sometimes feel excluded from the palpable solidarity reinforced by these social rituals.

There is a second insight offered by conflict theory. Cassell (1991) and Zola (1982) argue persuasively that those who are relegated to secondary status within society begin to engage in a type of internalized self-conflict. All people, regardless of ability or disability, are expected to conform to the internalized rules contained in societal norms (Goffman 1963). A person who experiences chronic illness may lose the chance to look like everyone else, but it is much less likely that she will lose the *inner desire* to be accepted like everyone else. Thus the disabled individual experiences the sense of powerlessness at both personal and intrapersonal levels. One who must cope with a life-changing illness must interpret activities from the past, find ways to deal with present activities and test hypotheses regarding what will work in the future (Karp 1996).

Insights from conflict theory can help us to understand how the stigma of chronic disease has both internal and external manifestations. If one accepts the premise that leisure draws on the full creative potential of each person, participation in leisure can become a source of healing. Conflict theory suggests that it is not enough to say that people with disabilities must have access to leisure. They must, in addition, be able to draw upon leisure experience as a means of directing their own personal growth and power.

Activity 14.6: Conflict perspective

Can you think of events in which you experience what it means to be a winner or loser? Have you ever felt alienated from group leisure activities?
  Describe how leisure is linked to feelings of power or powerlessness.

Interactionism

Through leisure, one is able to interact playfully with the serious business of living (Csikszentmihalyi 1993). Mead (1934) wrote extensively about the relationship of games and play to the socialized self. Although it is difficult to ascribe precise meanings to particular leisure acts, it is possible to speak symbolically about how this occurs. Leisure provides access to instruments, forms and symbols (Kelly & Godbey 1992). Consider, for example, dancing. In this activity, the body is used as an instrument, and movement becomes the vehicle for expression. The dance itself may take on many forms, from classical to ritual to improvised. The dancer in the act of dancing becomes a symbol, conveying meaning to others. This example attempts to illustrate how the participant, acting freely within the activity, is drawn into open expression of subjective meaning. What remains unseen, and can therefore be known only intuitively, is that through this self-generated expression, the person participates in his or her own development.

Within the boundaries of leisure, time and action are under control of the individual. Time can be treasured, planned for, avoided or enjoyed. All actions are controlled by the individual who experiences, through the very act itself, meaning, self-realization, the release of energy and spiritual renewal. From a symbolic perspective, leisure incorporates the elements of control, attitude and experience, through which the boundaries of actual time and space are transcended and new meaning is made (Bundy & Canella 1994). However, the meaning of leisure transcends the individual actor or player. The social values and meanings constructed by individuals within a particular society or a particular segment of society achieve external expression through predominant patterns of leisure (Dumazedier 1967).

Activity 14.7: Symbolic interaction perspective

How might your pattern of leisure participation serve as a metaphor for things that you value? How do you experience leisure as improvised performance?

A POSTMODERN PERSPECTIVE

In thinking about leisure and postmodernity, we must also consider how leisure has come to be perceived within a specific time period (mid- to late twentieth century) as the excesses of modernity have become more obvious. Post-modernism's viewpoint can be characterized by the need to experience individual meaning within popular culture shaped by mass consumption (Kelly & Godbey 1992). Modern society is one in which consumption devalues the 'pure' impulse for play (Jarvie & Maguire 1994). It is also one in which the boundaries between play and work have become increasingly blurred (Rojek 1995).

Just as no single classical theory was adequate to describe leisure's multifaceted nature, so too no single postmodern approach works well. One insight offered by a postmodern approach is that through affirming the existence of multiple ways of expression within occupational forms such as leisure, we come to recognize and embrace the diversity of human experience. A second insight is that the choice afforded in leisure creates a bridge between the traditional and the modern, the personal and the public, the secular and the sacred. In choosing, we balance the intricate relationship between individual needs and social forms.

Activity 14.8: Postmodern perspective

In what way does your leisure balance the traditional and the modern, the secular and the sacred?

MULTIDIMENSIONAL PERSPECTIVES

It should be clear from the preceding discussion that the complexity of leisure calls for a multi-dimensional orientation. Early research into leisure tended to focus on how people are socialized into particular patterns of participation (Cutler & Hendricks 1990). Drawing on the work of Marx and Weber, sociologists probed the effects of class, gender, race, age and socioeconomic status on leisure preference and participation. Many of these early studies have been criticized because they overlooked the symbolic nature of leisure and because they used cross-sectional rather than longitudinal methods (Cutler & Hendricks 1990). However, from this early research has emerged

a continuing interest in patterns of participation as they occur across the lifespan.

Another benefit of early studies is the insight that the unconstrained choice evident in leisure offers opportunities for both normal and pathological engagement. Deviant behaviour in leisure can take many forms, including workaholism, addiction, compulsiveness, frenetic activity and even frenetic exercise (Kelly & Godbey 1992).

Most recently, social scientists have focused less on pathological expressions of leisure than on the continuity of participation patterns across the lifespan (Cutler & Hendricks 1990). The grandmother sitting in the front garden may feel joy in watching her grandson playing on a swing, remembering what the experience felt like. It is not necessary for both persons take part in the swinging activity to share the meaning attached to it.

Kelly's continuum for leisure activity

Kelly (1978) was among the first sociologists to propose that leisure patterns could be discerned by combining the viewpoint of the actor with its relationship to social structures. He identified five common leisure elements and four basic leisure types.

Leisure elements

Kelly (1978) proposed that participation contained five key elements, each of which exists on a continuum:

- intensity (passive to active)
- sociability (solitary to large group)
- spontaneity (impromptu to highly ritualized)
- location (private space to public space)
- absorption (mind-focused to total mind and body).

These elements, observed in all types of leisure forms, create a way of classifying engagement. The student who takes a break from studying by playing a computer game is engaging in solitary activity that is mentally absorbing and in which she may be the only player or one of many players existing in cyberspace. Another student, attending a country dance group, is engaged in a group activity that is held in a public place, scheduled and ritualized as well as intensely physical.

Leisure types

Building on his concepts of leisure continua, Kelly (1983) identified four basic leisure types:

- unconditional
- compensatory
- relational
- role-determined.

Activities are unconditional when they call forth the spontaneous improvisation and playfulness of the participant. Opportunities for self-expression are central to this type of leisure. Activities are considered compensatory when the participant uses them for relaxation or stress release. In these activities, the differences between 'pure' work and 'pure' recreation are highlighted. Activities are relational when they call for a high degree of spontaneous social interaction between participants. Going to parties or rock concerts might be identified as activities typical of this category. Activities are role-determined when they are part of a larger role-set for the individual. Social behaviour during the activity is often constrained by norms or mores. Good examples are a family wedding or a social event for company employees.

Although in his recent writings Kelly has stated that all attempts to model leisure are premature (Kelly & Godbey 1992), the conceptual linkage between chosen activities and social roles is central to the study of leisure as occupation.

A developmental model

An alternative conceptual scheme for understanding types of leisure is offered by B. G. Gunter and Nancy Gunter (1980). Recognizing the influence of life circumstances on leisure participation, the authors outline a life-context approach that recognizes the effect of space, time and lifestyle on leisure choice (Table 14.1). Dumazedier's (1967) concept of freedom is used by the Gunters in model development, but it is amplified to suggest that certain aspects of lifestyles influence the choices that people make. Leisure lifestyles can be differentiated from each other by the relative pleasure a person derives from free time and by the way in which that time is used.

For example, the mother of young children may feel alienated from pure leisure experiences that she once enjoyed. As the children grow, she may take pleasure through institutional participation in sport, school or religious activities;

Table 14.1 Gunter & Gunter's leisure styles framework

Type of leisure	Type of time use	Examples
Pure leisure	Time planned for pleasure	Creative outlets Hobbies Holidays, vacations
Anomic leisure	Time on one's hands	Alienated youth Unemployed Empty nest Disengaged retirees
Institutional leisure	Time devoted to others	Work related Family related Volunteer work Religious practice Social causes
Alienated leisure	Time bind	Underemployed Role overload Burn out

she may engage in few leisure pursuits on her own. When the children leave home, she may feel the need to fill her time by resuming old hobbies or developing new interests. At the same time, she may still enjoy types of leisure in which she engaged while her children were young.

A major advantage of the Gunters' approach is that it assumes a lifespan perspective toward leisure engagement. At its root is the recognition that, throughout life, people use time, space, material objects and other human beings to create their own perceptions of coherence and meaning. These roles and identities are not static: they are always being modified in response to life experiences, which can themselves also be modified by the therapeutic process. The opportunities offered by leisure for free expression and self-fulfilment make the occupational form of leisure a natural therapeutic tool.

LEISURE AND OCCUPATIONAL THERAPY

While social scientists study leisure for a myriad of reasons, occupational therapists have a rather single-minded concern. Leisure is an important lifelong occupation. Nelson (1988) has defined the relationship between occupational form, or the set of circumstances within which the person performs, and occupational performance, which is, of course, the doing of the action or activity itself.

We have seen that Dumazedier's (1967) definition of leisure comprises two parts. Leisure is (1) a freely chosen activity that (2) enhances the self in a number of potential ways. These include (but are not limited to) relaxation, diversion, the broadening of knowledge, spontaneous social participation and the free use of creative potential.

If we accept Dumazedier's definition or some variation thereof, it will have many potential implications for practice. First, this definition can change the way in which we think about leisure for ourselves and for our clients. Leisure is more than activity that fills up time not allotted to

'serious' work. It is certainly more complex than the words of the American Occupational Therapy Association's (1994, p. 12) uniform terminology might suggest:

planning and participating in play or leisure activities. Maintaining a balance of play or leisure activities with work and productive activities, and activities of daily living. Obtaining, utilizing, and maintaining equipment and supplies.

It is more complex even than described by Davidson (1991, pp. 162–163) in a major textbook on occupational therapy:

Throughout the lifetime, a person needs a time away from work and responsibilities, a time to restore oneself and find meaning in life. The term *leisure* is commonly used for this activity. Leisure is characterized by relative choice and is usually shared by people of like interests. The activity may be something one likes to do alone or with other people. … The social mood is usually one of playfulness and one that is relatively free from standards and rules (although religious and sports occasions may involve a great many rules specific to those groups). … The settings are those away from work and away from the management of the home or personal living situation.

In leisure, we both express who we are and become who we are (Kelly & Godbey 1992). Leisure is central to our life, not separate from it; it fulfils important needs not met in any other form of occupation. It is therefore necessary to adopt a more encompassing definition of leisure for our practice, to serve as a guideline for both assessment and intervention with individual clients.

APPLYING DUMAZEDIER'S DEFINITION

In order for an activity to reflect Dumazedier's (1967) definition of leisure, it must be freely chosen and must yield benefits important to the individual. In order to understand the implications of this definition to our clients, both these concepts require further discussion.

Freely-chosen activity

That an activity be freely chosen is the most commonly listed criterion of leisure. In the spirit of Tom Sawyer, work is what a person *must* do, while play and leisure are what he *wants* to do. However, work and leisure do not represent a simple dichotomy (Primeau 1996). Any activity can be freely chosen. Thus so long as it also meets the other criteria, any activity can be leisure. Furthermore, one can create play and leisure within the context of work or self-care activities. For example, Primeau (1996) described parents and their pre-school aged children who embedded play within household chores. Other authors have described play that occurs between co-workers during staff meetings or individuals who were able to turn the most boring of assembly line tasks into activities in which they could become totally involved (Csikszentmihalyi 1993).

For Kelly & Godbey (1992), self-determination, rather than the absence of limits or constraints, is the most critical aspect of freedom within a leisure activity. Self-determination and the freedom to choose are aspects of a larger construct: internal control. In their discussions of play or leisure, some authors (Bundy & Canella 1994, Neumann 1971) have listed control, rather than simply the freedom to choose, as the factor that determines whether or not an experience is play or leisure. Within the broad construct of internal control also appear such factors as matching challenges to skills, determining outcomes and optimal levels of choice within an activity (Bundy & Canella 1994).

Consider Amy, a 41-year-old divorced woman who was becoming seriously involved with a new partner. Her partner, Alex, was an avid member of a wheelchair tennis team. Alex invited Amy to join the women's team and to play in an upcoming tournament. Amy was both thrilled and excited at the same time. She wanted to share Alex's interests and she loved sports, but this activity was more strenuous and challenging than any she had ever tried before. There were moments (straining to sustain a rally, trying to stay calm during a serve) when she did not feel at all in control. At those times, the experience could hardly be called leisure.

Rarely is an individual in total control of any activity or event; in fact, total control is not likely to be desirable. When, as is common, a leisure activity is shared with another individual, control must also be shared (Neumann 1971). At the most basic level, each participant must retain at least enough freedom to take part in, or discontinue, the activity at will.

Consider Margaret, a 50-year-old woman full of fears and anger. Margaret would only engage in activities in which she believed she could have total control. She would accept invitations to card games or board games only if she was sure she could win. Needless to say, Margaret's family and friends resented her behaviour, but they felt that they needed to protect her weak ego. A bridge game that looked like 'leisure' was really a great deal of 'work' for her family.

Benefits of leisure

Through leisure, individuals freely use their creative potential to invent something of who they are and who they aim to be. The benefits are both immediate and long term. They include relaxation, diversion, spontaneous social participation, broadening of knowledge and the free use of creative potential. Although not listed explicitly, another important benefit of leisure – pleasure – seems to be implied (Csikszentmihalyi 1975).

Leisure activities are clearly complex; many different benefits can come from a single activity. However, many activities of different types may be necessary to reap *all* the benefits of leisure. Furthermore, the benefits listed by Dumazedier do not appear to be of the same order. For example, Kleiber (1985) indicated that diversion (or disengagement) was necessary. That is, if an individual is to experience leisure or any of its benefits, she must disengage temporarily from the real or perceived constraints of daily life (e.g. pain, poor health or family demands).

Consider Leon, a 28-year-old man with intractable pain associated with a brain tumour. Despite significant physical limitations, Leon enjoys many active sports, including skiing. However, the high mountain altitudes often increase his pain and have occasionally resulted in seizures. After discussing this problem with his family, he decided to accompany them on hill walks. This change gave him access to the outdoors without taxing his resources or those of his family.

Similarly, although Dumazedier (1967) lists the free use of creative potential as a benefit of leisure, the importance that authors such as Kelly & Godbey (1992) place on the *relationships* between creativity and leisure suggest that it is a necessary component as much as a benefit of leisure. In all discussions of creativity and leisure, there is heavy emphasis on its *free* use. While rules are a part of leisure activities (e.g. sports), they are meant to inform the actions of the player rather than to constrain her creativity (Caillois 1979). Nonetheless, some individuals will feel too constrained in activities such as organized sports and will need to seek other or additional leisure outlets for their creativity.

When one seeks relaxation as a benefit of leisure, it is presumably with the intent of restoring wholeness to mind, body and spirit. This implies that not all activities that have relaxation as an end product can be classified as leisure. Kelly & Godbey described both leisure and recreation as requiring action. They note that it 'may be physical, intellectual, communicative, imaginative, contemplative, creative, habitual, emotional or some combination of elements' (1992, p. 19).

Leisure undoubtedly involves action in the most inclusive sense, but it does involve action. While they may provide relaxation, napping and sleeping are not leisure; much film- and television-watching may also fall under this rubric. Douglas & Johnson (cited in Kelly & Godbey 1992, p. 204) lumped these expressions of 'leisure' together with drug use, pornography and other forms of indulgence:

Such experiences are designed to produce a feeling of gratification without the cost or risk of real action. Just because they may offer a feeling of freedom, they may stand in the way of the exercise of freedom. They are unauthentic because they are deceptive. Play becomes an escape rather than initiative and action. Leisure reduced to mental state may be the basis of self-deception and bondage rather than an act of freedom.

Activity 14.9

Would you agree with Douglas & Johnson, or does their position simply reflect a particular set of values?

When we ask clients about their leisure, we must evaluate their answers for the presence of action. However, before concluding that an activity does not meet the criteria for leisure because it does not involve action, we must be certain that our definition of action is broad enough. That is, action is not always physical.

Dumazedier (1967) listed spontaneous social participation as an important benefit of leisure. Kelly & Godbey (1992) described leisure as fundamentally social. They indicated that, because 'the interaction is the action', the most significant factor in judging the success of many leisure events is who is there. Who sat beside me at dinner? Who danced with me? Who drove home with me? While participation and interaction are the benefits, the challenge of leisure is communication. Social communication in a leisure context may be particularly tricky; a wide variety of play may be taking place at one time (Kelly & Godbey 1992). To successfully reap the social benefits associated with leisure, an individual must be able to read the cues of the situation, that is, to understand how he should behave toward others. He also must be able to give clear cues that tell others how they should behave toward him (Bateson 1971).

While many leisure activities are carried out with others, some are solitary. However, even when leisure occurs alone, it has social consequences. Leisure influences who individuals are and who they are becoming (Bundy & Canella 1994). Those newly created individuals, in turn, assume other roles in day-to-day life. Thus, leisure activities provide one with the opportunity to become more able or to develop a new dimension of selfhood (Kelly & Godbey 1992). In a related way, Dumazedier (1967) listed broadening one's knowledge as a benefit of leisure.

As we learn ourselves who we are, we also teach others and learn from them about who they are. Plato is reputed to have said he could learn more about another in an hour of play than in a year of conversation. That alone is reason enough for therapists to promote leisure with their clients.

Individuals who experience a disability stand to attain the same benefits from leisure *after* the disability as before. That is, through participation in leisure, they can teach both themselves and others about a new self. Depending on the individual, the revealing nature of leisure can be either an incentive or a deterrent to participation. Therapists must explore in a sensitive fashion the ways in which leisure-related identity statements of individuals have been altered after a disability.

ASSESSMENT ISSUES

Before beginning an assessment of leisure, it is necessary to understand the individual's perception of the value of leisure in general. There is a real difference between the young man who has skied avidly since the age of 7 and who cannot imagine not skiing and the 67-year-old farmer who believes that all leisure is a foolish waste of time. In both cases, the assessment of leisure is likely to be important. However, the language one uses in the assessment will be critical. Elsewhere (Bundy & Canella 1994), I have relayed the story of a woman who thought my questions about play to be a waste of time. However, when I asked her about 'activities in which she became totally involved, forgetting everything else', she told a wonderful story of rug-weaving.

Even under the best of circumstances, the assessment of leisure with a client is not easy. There is no perfect instrument that captures all the relevant aspects. Thus one must use several scales and methodologies to piece the entire puzzle together.

The types and meaningfulness of activities in which an individual engages (or engaged in the past) provide a part of the picture. Two complementary assessments published in occupational therapy literature – the Activity Index (Revised) (Gregory 1983) and the Meaningfulness of Activity Scale (Gregory 1983) – can shed light on this area. However, therapists should be aware that these scales were created for use with retirees, and, even then, they provide only a partial list of potential leisure activities. Kelly & Godbey (1992) indicated that much of the most highly valued leisure occurs within the context of daily life, but that unless individuals are prompted,

they do not think of these activities. Thus, even though the Activity Index contains blanks for additional activities, individuals may not think to list them.

Although it is possible to derive a score from these scales, the interpretation may not be easy. Bundy (1993) poses the question of whether it is more desirable for an individual to be interested in many activities or to have intense involvement in only a few. Furthermore, the scores from both assessments represent ordinal rather than interval data. Because of this, it is unlikely that scores, for example, of '(1) do not enjoy it at all', '(2) enjoy doing it very little', and '(3) enjoy doing it somewhat' represent equal intervals. Thus adding them together does not create a meaningful score.

The Leisure Diagnostic Battery (LDB) (Witt & Ellis 1989) provides information regarding leisure in the following areas: perceived freedom, perceived barriers, preferences and knowledge of leisure opportunities. While the LDB provides valuable information and has, for the most part, shown promise with regard to reliability and validity, it also is subject to serious criticism and must be used with caution.

The use of the word 'recreation' in questions (e.g. 'I usually have fun when I'm involved in recreation activities') may lead individuals to think only about sports and other organized activities rather than also including more day-to-day leisure experiences. Further, the LDB is scored on a 3-point Likert scale, reflecting the degree to which an item reflects the preference of the individual; the points are summed to create a score. Again, the data are ordinal and cannot be added meaningfully.

Much of the information that an occupational therapist needs for intervention planning must be gathered by interview. As indicated, whether one uses the term 'leisure' in the course of an interview depends on the person. There is no existing structured interview that yields all the information we seek, so each therapist must create the questions to capture the information that he or she needs. Following the structure provided by Dumazedier (1967), one might seek information in four overlapping areas: freedom to choose (or the broader category of internal control), ability to disengage from the constraints of day-to-day life, the use of creativity (especially the opportunity to be and become) and benefits or ways in which the self is enhanced (e.g. relaxation, broadening of knowledge or spontaneous social participation).

INTERVENTION ISSUES

In leisure, as in all life activities, an individual needs occasions to do and become that which is most meaningful to her or him. Leisure is an important avenue by which that occurs; it is a significant lifelong occupation.

Many things can prevent an individual becoming involved in leisure, especially following an injury or debilitating illness. Some of those are reasonably easy to address. Consider, for example, Ralph who, prior to a spinal injury that left him paraplegic, had run 6–10 miles a day. Ralph described that he ran because he wanted to keep fit, but something in his tone of voice suggested that it was more than that. He did not run simply out of fear of getting fat; he ran because he loved it. How could Ralph, who no longer had movement or sensation below the waist, replace running? It was simple. He began wheelchair road racing. 'I could go out and push 10 or 20 miles a night and kind of feel the same, you know, level of satisfaction.' By talking with people like Ralph, it is possible to uncover the benefits they get from cherished leisure activities and help them to replace those activities or regain the ability to do them in another way.

The greatest barrier to participation in leisure is not physical: it involves one's belief system. Pieper (cited in Kelly & Godbey 1992) suggested that it is spiritual. He believed that leisure was a way of joyfully affirming one's place in the universe. Some people, Pieper believed, could not obtain leisure. They were 'incapable of accepting their lives in the world with joy, and were therefore, incapable of accepting all the good things

to be found in their culture or of experiencing leisure' (p. 180).

Take, for example, the case of Rose, a 44-year-old woman who had 'done the drug scene' for much of her early adult life. She was always high. She was always surrounded by people because she was afraid to be alone and face herself. One day, after taking a drug dose large enough to kill her, Rose decided that she wanted to live. She finished college; she developed many meaningful relationships. Despite rheumatoid arthritis and a significant visual impairment, Rose lives in the mountains where she loves camping, feeding the birds and watching the deer in her garden. Rose has become an advocate for women and people with disabilities. Although she describes her political involvement as paying a 'debt to society', one suspects that she also loves the social interactions that these activities afford (Lewis, in preparation).

Helping an individual to make the kind of transition that Rose made in her life can be extremely difficult. Helping others to acquire leisure may just be a simple matter of adapting an activity or helping them see the possibilities and make the connections. Sometimes it is much more difficult, helping an individual to see the reasons she has to celebrate. Rose developed a passion for life. An important part of that passion was doing things for the pure joy of it.

CONCLUSION

In this chapter, we have explored some of the difficulties of defining leisure and highlighted the importance of taking a multifaceted view. We have looked at the importance for occupational therapists of thinking about the meaning of leisure. It is all too easy to think of leisure in simple terms: of its being simply the third division of human occupation after self-care and productivity. Sociology can help us to understand and analyse the complexity of this topic.

REFERENCES

American Occupational Therapy Association 1994 Uniform terminology for occupational therapy, 3rd edn. American Occupational Therapy Association, Rockville, MD

Bateson G 1971 The message, 'this is play'. In: Herron R E, Sutton-Smith B (eds) Child's play. John Wiley, New York

Bundy A C 1993 Assessment of play and leisure: delineation of the problem. American Journal of Occupational Therapy 47: 217–222

Bundy A C, Canella J M 1994 Leisure. In: Bonder B R, Wagner M B (eds) Functional performance in older adults. F A Davis, Philadelphia

Caillois R 1979 Man, play, and games. Schocken, New York

Cassell E J 1991 The nature of suffering. Oxford University Press, New York

Csikszentmihalyi M 1975 Beyond boredom and anxiety. Jossey-Bass, San Francisco

Csikszentmihalyi M 1993 The evolving self: a psychology for the third millennium. Harper Collins, New York

Cutler S J, Hendricks J 1990 Leisure and time use across the life course. In: Binstock R H and George L K (eds) Handbook of aging and the social sciences, 3rd edn. Academic Press, New York

Davidson H 1991 Performance and the social environment. In: Christiansen C, Baum C (eds) Occupational therapy: overcoming human performance deficits. Slack, Thorofare, NJ

Dumazedier J 1967 Toward a society of leisure. Free Press, New York

Durkheim E 1893 [1984] The division of labor in society. Free Press, New York

Goffman E 1963 Stigma: notes on the management of a spoiled identity. Simon & Schuster, New York

Gregory M D 1983 Occupational behavior and life satisfaction among retirees. American Journal of Occupational Therapy 37: 533–548

Gunter B G, Gunter N C 1980 Leisure styles: a conceptual framework for modern leisure. Sociological Quarterly 21: 361–374

Jarvie G, Maguire J 1994 Sport and leisure in social thought. Routledge, London

Karp D A 1996 Speaking of sadness: depression, disconnection, and the meaning of illness. Oxford University Press, New York

Kelly J R 1978 Leisure styles and choices in three environments. Pacific Sociological Review 21: 187–207

Kelly J R 1983 Leisure identities and interactions. George Allen & Unwin, London

Kelly J R, Godbey G 1992 The sociology of leisure. Venture Publishing. State College, PA.

Kleiber D A 1985 Motivational reorientation in adulthood and the resource of leisure. In: Kleiber D A, Maehr M L (eds) Advances in motivation and achievement, vol. 4. JAI Press, Greenwich, CT

Lewis A (in preparation) Motivations for leisure. Master's thesis, Colorado State University

Luschen G, Sage GH 1981 Sport in sociological perspective. In: Luschen G, Sage G H (eds) Handbook of social science of sport. Stipes, Champaign, IL

Mead G H 1934 Mind, self, and society. University of Chicago Press, Chicago

Nelson D 1988 Occupation: form and performance. American Journal of Occupational Therapy 42: 633–641

Neulinger J 1981 The psychology of leisure: research approaches to the study of leisure. Charles C. Thomas, Springfield, IL

Neumann E A 1971 The elements of play. MSS Information, New York

Primeau L 1996 Work and leisure: transcending the dichotomy. American Journal of Occupational Therapy 50: 569–577

Rojek C 1995 Decentring leisure: rethinking leisure theory. Sage, London

Veblen T 1899 [1965] The theory of the leisure class. A M Kelley, New York

Witt P A, Ellis G 1989 The leisure diagnostic battery user's manual. North Texas State University, Denton, TX

Zola I K 1982 Missing pieces: a chronicle of living with a disability. Temple University Press, Philadelphia, PA

15

Normalization and critical disability theory

Kirsten Stalker   Chris Jones

INTRODUCTION

The purpose of this chapter is first to outline some important developments in theoretical thinking about disability over recent years, and second, to examine the implications of these for occupational therapy. In the first part of the chapter, two main areas will be discussed. The first is normalization, the most influential philosophy driving services for people with learning difficulties today. A brief outline will also be given of person-centred planning, which is a relatively new development derived, but different, from normalization. The second main topic is the social model of disability, developed by people with physical/sensory impairments, which is having a radical effect on the way in which disability is conceived and understood. Reference will also be made to more 'individualizing' models of disability, although these have been largely rejected by disabled people as theoretically flawed and politically oppressive.

In the same way that normalization has had its greatest impact in the field of learning difficulties, so the social model of disability has been most influential in relation to people with physical and sensory impairment. Both theories would support a 'collective' or inclusive view of disability, but in practice, as we shall see, normalization has not found favour with people with physical/sensory impairment, while the relevance of the social model to people with learning difficulties has, to date, hardly been explored. In the second part of the chapter, the implications of these theoretical developments for occupational therapy will be explored with particular reference to learning difficulties.

Throughout the chapter, the term 'learning difficulties' is used rather than such others as 'mental retardation', 'learning disability' or 'intellectual impairment'. This is the preferred term of organizations of people with learning difficulties in the UK.

NORMALIZATION

Whitehead (1992) traces the origins of normalization to a number of wider post-war political and sociological developments:

- the human and civil rights movements
- the challenge to structural functionalism coming from labelling and deviancy theories
- the emergence of the welfare state.

It was, however, in Scandinavia that the concept was born.

Scandinavian origins

Normalization was first formulated by Nirje (1969) and Bank-Mikkelson (1980), its principles being enshrined in Swedish law in 1967, at a time when many people with learning difficulties were living out their lives in bleak long-stay institutions. The main concern of this early form of normalization was to develop services in such a way as to enable people with learning difficulties to enjoy 'patterns of life and conditions of everyday living which are as close as possible to the regular circumstances and ways of life of society' (Nirje 1980, p. 33).

It was emphasized, for example, that people should have the right to experience the same sort of daily and weekly routines, age-appropriate activities, heterosexual (sic) relationships, economic standards and level of self-determination as the rest of the population. There was some difference between the Danish and Swedish 'versions', the former emphasizing the importance of outcome, that is, the achievement of a lifestyle for people with learning difficulties similar to that of non-disabled people, the latter focusing more

on process, i.e. the means by which this goal might be attained. A process orientation would, for example, focus on setting up services that would offer people 'ordinary' patterns of daily life. In both cases, at this stage in its development, 'normalization' amounted to a series of principles that were intended to shape service delivery but which did not add up to a coherent theoretical framework (Emerson 1992).

Radicalization of the concept by Wolfensberger

The idea was developed and radicalized by Wolf Wolfensberger in the USA. He redefined normalization as:

the utilisation of means which are as culturally normative as possible, in order to establish and / or maintain personal behaviour and characteristics which are as culturally normative as possible. (Wolfensberger 1972, p. 28)

Wolfensberger exposed the powerful role of ideology in colouring people's thoughts and behaviour, and the often 'unconscious' nature of what he called 'bad' ideologies. Racial discrimination, for example, is quoted as a manifestation of unconscious ideology since most people profess a belief in equality. Similarly, the so-called caring professions, or human management services, have the declared aim of giving humane care and treatment, but, in reality, they often segregate and 'dehumanize' people.

Activity 15.1

From your fieldwork experience, can you identify examples of segregating or dehumanizing practices?

Drawing on deviancy theory (see Chapter 9), Wolfensberger accounted for this contradiction between beliefs and action in terms of the 'stigma' attached to people seen as significantly different from others in some negative (or 'devalued') way. He stressed the cultural nature of such judgments, since certain attributes (such as obesity in women) are valued in some countries but denigrated in others. People viewed as deviant are liable to be cast, *en masse*, into certain social roles, those with learning difficulties having been seen variously as subhuman, menaces, objects of ridicule, eternal children and so on. Society can respond to perceived deviancy by destroying, segregating, reversing or preventing it. Wolfensberger is concerned with the last two of these. Because deviancy lies 'in the eye of the beholder', he argues, the most effective way of reversing or preventing it is to ensure that individuals with learning difficulties minimize those attributes or behaviours likely to be viewed as deviant, and maximize or develop those which are socially desirable. Following some criticism (see below) of the emphasis on 'normality' in his work, Wolfensberger (1983) proposed that the term 'normalization' be replaced by 'social role valorization', thereby stressing the importance of people with learning difficulties occupying socially valued roles within their communities.

Wolfensberger stressed that, at policy and practice level, normalization inevitably goes hand-in-hand with social integration. Indeed, there can be no doubt that normalization has had a major positive effect on the nature and quality of service provision, not only for people with learning difficulties. By helping to raise awareness of the empty lives led by many people in segregated institutions, and the subsequent damaging emotional and psychological effects, the ethos of normalization has been an important influence on the development of community care policies for all people who use services.

Theoretical weaknesses

Despite its positive elements, there are serious criticisms to be made of some of the underlying implications of normalization. As outlined above, Wolfensberger contends that, in order to promote their integration in, and acceptance by, the community at large, people with learning difficulties should attempt to 'blend in' by being as 'ordinary', conventional and unobtrusive as possible. This emphasis on conformity leaves little room for variation and diversity, either at the level of individual taste or preference, or at a sociocultural level, be it in terms of race,

gender, sexual orientation or indeed any other significant dimension. In this sense, normalization can, ironically, be seen as itself devaluing disabled people. The insistence, for example, on the importance of associating with non-disabled people seems to imply that it is undesirable for people with learning difficulties to associate with each other. It has also been pointed out that, by exhorting people with learning difficulties to adopt the views and values of the *status quo*, normalization expects them to take on the perspective of the very people who are devaluing them (Smith & Brown 1992).

Normalization pays little, if any, attention to the economic and social factors that account for so many of the barriers facing disadvantaged people. For example, people with learning difficulties do not enjoy the same access to educational, training and employment opportunities as others. Many have extremely low incomes, often relying on welfare benefits. In addition, certain features of modern Western society, such as the value placed on 'quick-wittedness', the primacy of the written word and sophisticated technology may act as considerable barriers to inclusion for many people. Normalization does not take account of these structural factors and can thus be seen as an inherently conservative philosophy. As Smith & Brown (1992) point out, it now needs to be developed in line with current notions of empowerment.

O'Brien's five accomplishments

Much of Wolfensberger's work is presented in a dense, theoretical style that lessens its accessibility. In contrast, John O'Brien's accounts of normalization are generally presented in a relatively simple and straightforward manner. Furthermore, O'Brien has restated the importance of individual choice and control. He has written extensively on advocacy and social inclusion, and is best known for setting out the 'five service accomplishments' (1987), targets at which community services should aim if they are to enact the principles of normalization (Box 15.1). O'Brien describes the five accomplishments as 'a definition of the principle of normalization'.

Box 15.1 O'Brien's five service accomplishments	
Community presence	Meaning that people with learning difficulties should make use of ordinary, mainstream facilities
Choice	Whereby people should have support in making their own choices both at a day-to-day level and about major life events
Competence	Creating opportunities for people to reach their full potential by developing a range of skills
Respect	Which refers to people's right to occupy a valued role within a network of reciprocal roles
Community participation	Which means the importance of being part of a growing network of friends

Person-centred planning

The five accomplishments form the basis of various different approaches to supporting individuals in planning their own futures. Person-centred planning, developed in North America by O'Brien, Herb Lovett, Jack Pierpoint and Marsha Forest among others, is a term used to denote a variety of related approaches to planning while also promoting inclusive practices within local communities. It is based on an explicit value system that places the person at the centre of the process, emphasizes the importance of 'respect for the dignity and completeness' of that person and 'a celebration of individuals' uniqueness' (O'Brien & Lovett 1992). Both in principle and in process, person-centred planning differs significantly from traditional methods of 'assessment', which are based on a particular perspective on disability and focus on professional judgment of need.

TRADITIONAL MODELS OF DISABILITY

For many years, professional policy and practice within the health and 'caring professions' has been dominated by the medical model of disability; some would argue that it still is. As its name implies, this model equates disability with chronic illness, ascribes a 'sick role' to the individual and focuses on physical 'dysfunction'. People are classified according to their particular medical condition, diagnosis or impairment. From this perspective, the appropriate professional response is aimed at improving the individual's physical or functional capacities, the limitations or perceived inadequacies of which are seen as the sole cause of any difficulties. The medical model is part of an individualizing frame of reference that includes:

- psychodynamic theory
- the personal tragedy model
- the administrative model.

When viewed from the perspective of psychodynamic theory, the experience of being or becoming disabled is assumed to constitute a continuing personal tragedy, triggering a grief reaction in the same way that a bereavement would do. It is up to the individual to adapt to both the tragedy and to society (Oliver 1990).

Certain individuals may be judged to have had outstanding success in overcoming the odds against them, thus attaining the status of 'hero'. More probably, however, disabled people are in constant mourning for their lost or missing 'wholeness'. This 'variant' has been described as the personal tragedy model (Hevey 1993).

The administrative model of disability (Finkelstein 1993) is particularly relevant for occupational therapists. Here, disabled people become subject to endless professional and bureaucratic intervention, ostensibly in order to administer to their psychological, emotional and practical needs. In reality, however, the professions have another agenda – to establish and maintain for themselves the power, prestige and financial rewards associated with professional status (see Chapter 12). This process serves to perpetuate the dependency and powerlessness of disabled people. Abberley (1995) sets out how he sees this dynamic working in relation to occupational therapy. He suggests that therapists tend to take credit for successful interventions but not responsibility when therapy fails. An important distinction between the medical model and the others identified above is, of course, that the former was developed, and would be defended, by many professionals (and perhaps some others), whereas both the personal tragedy and the administrative models have been identified by disabled people as critiques of the *status quo*. The most influential analysis to date, developed by disabled people, is the social model.

Activity 15.2

Make a note of your reaction to what you have just read – does it surprise you? Does it conflict with what you have been taught so far? Discuss your thoughts in a small group, and then read on.

SOCIAL MODEL OF DISABILITY

In his seminal volume on the social model of disability, Oliver (1990) discusses the different meanings attached to impairment across cultures and across centuries. Drawing on Gwaltney (1970), for example, he shows how the prevalence of blindness among inhabitants of a Mexican village was viewed as a result of divine intervention, and those thus affected were treated with special respect. It was seen as an issue for the community rather than for individuals. Similarly, Ryan & Thomas (1987) record that, in certain Alpine villages where the incidence of learning disability was high owing to deficiencies in the water, those affected were seen as 'angels', a gift from God, and families who did not have a member with learning difficulties were shunned. Unlike Wolfensberger, however, Oliver has no interest in suggesting that such attitudes arise from unconscious processes; rather, having demonstrated that disability is not medicalized or individualized in every society, he then draws on a Marxist analysis to explain the oppression of disabled people within capitalist societies.

A Marxist analysis

During the rise of industrialism in Western societies, Oliver argues, disabled people came to be seen as a burden since they were generally unable to undertake the heavy physical labour required in factories and thus to contribute to the capitalist economy. They were subjected to harsh regimes in 'workhouses', along with impoverished older people and orphans, thus creating an enforced dependency that still exists today, albeit within a more 'humane' welfare framework. Again like Wolfensberger, Oliver pays attention to the role of ideology in relation to disability, but his interest lies in its construction of disability rather than (as in Wolfensberger's formulation) its interpretation of something whose actual existence is not in doubt. Within the social model, the definition of disability is an important issue.

Disability redefined

Disability has been defined in different ways depending on the perspective of the producer. The International Classification of Impairments, Disabilities and Handicaps (ICIDH), developed by the World Health Organisation, has been widely adopted and is currently used by the British Department of Health (Box 15.2).

This approach has, however, been criticized for its strongly medical focus and neglect of the social causes of disability. According to Oliver (1993), the ICIDH rests upon able-bodied assumptions of disability and [does] not accord with the personal realities of disabled people'. In contrast, the social model of disability points to the material constraints and barriers within society, rather than an individual's actual impairment,

---

Box 15.2 WHO classifications

Impairment	Any loss or abnormality of psychological, physiological or anatomical structure or function
Disability	Any restriction or lack (resulting from an impairment) of ability to perform an activity in the manner or within the range considered normal for a human being
Handicap	A disadvantage for a given individual, resulting from an impairment or disability that limits or prevents the fulfilment of a role (depending on age, sex and social cultural factors) for that individual

as the source of disability (Finkelstein 1980). The Union of the Physically Impaired Against Segregation (UPIAS, 1976, cited by Oliver 1990) defined disability as follows:

The disadvantage or restriction of activity caused by a contemporary social organisation which takes little or no account of people who have a physical impairment and thus excludes them from the mainstream of social activities.

Thus the social model places great emphasis on people's right to mainstream life opportunities such as education, training and employment. It is closely associated with the disability movement, which has developed a sophisticated analysis of the discrimination facing disabled people, particularly in relation to transport, education, employment, access and income level (Barnes 1991).

> ### Activity 15.3
>
> Find out what legislation exists which is aimed at overcoming some of the discrimination noted in the text.

The place of impairment

Aspects of the social model have been challenged, however, and there are increasingly dissenting voices from within the disability movement itself. It is argued that the emphasis on 'disability' within the social model has led to a serious and detrimental underestimation of the significance of impairment. French (1993), while believing that most of the difficulties she faces as a visually impaired person are amenable to 'social' or environmental solutions, argues that this is not true of all problems arising from her impairment, citing as an example the difficulty of reading other people's non-verbal cues. She provides a helpful distinction between impairment and disability, noting that:

blindness is an impairment but lack of access to written information is a disability – a socially determined state of affairs which could be solved with more extensive Braille production, more money to pay for 'readers' and the greater use of taped material. (French 1993, p. 17)

Shakespeare & Watson (1995) also criticize disability theory for being 'shallow and simplistic'. While accepting the political reasons for focusing on disability and people's collective experience of discrimination, they argue that it is now time to consider the significance of the diversity of individual experience. They draw a parallel between 'early wave' feminism and disability theory: the concept of the term 'gender' allowed for the identification of the social construction of masculine and feminine roles, as opposed to the notion of male and female bodies, in much the same way as disability, as opposed to impairment, is used in the social model. In both cases, the authors argue, the body, and the idea of difference being located in the body, has been ignored. More recently, feminism has taken account of this notion of difference, allowing for consideration of both ideological construct and lived experience. Shakespeare & Watson argue that a similar shift needs to take place within disability theory, exploring the significance of difference and 'addressing disabled people's experience in terms of the body'.

Crow (1995), on the other hand, takes a rather different view of the social mode, arguing that it does not neglect impairment but instead has been misinterpreted. Crow identifies three dimensions of impairment:

- its physical manifestation
- an individual's subjective experience of it
- the impact upon it of the wider social context.

Calling for a 'renewal' of the social model, she argues for the need to focus on both disability *and* impairment, and the circumstances in which their causes and effects may interact.

A feminist perspective

A further criticism that has been made of the social model is its neglect of gender and race (Begum 1992, Morris 1992). Morris (1992) argues, at the same time, that *feminist* theory and research have generally excluded the experience of disabled women. A particularly telling example of this is the work of feminists such as Finch (1984) and Dalley (1988) on female carers. Having documented the stresses and strains to which many carers were subject, and the extent to which their lives were restricted by the demands of caring, these authors concluded that the best solution would be to set up some form of small-scale communal establishments in which older, frail and/or disabled people would live alongside non-disabled people, paid to be there, but with everyone supporting and helping each other according to their abilities. Dalley formulated this rather vague and unlikely vision without talking to disabled women (or men) to see what they thought of it, or indeed exploring their wider views and experiences of 'being cared for' and of caring (since there are also disabled carers, particularly among older women). Morris points out that most disabled people want, and have the right, to determine their own lifestyles and to live as independently as possible in their own home.

Begum (1992) points out that disability theory has neglected the experiences of disabled women (including black disabled women), tending to see disabled people as an homogeneous group with no gender difference. This may be explained by the fact that the social model has been generated largely by (white) men. Begum argues that both disability and gender are socially constructed and that the impact of each on the individual will vary depending on the extent to which he or she can be associated with some other, differently valued, social group. Begum argues that 'the concerns of disabled women strike at the core of the disability rights and feminist movements' (1992, p. 61). She identifies three issues central to a feminist analysis of the social position of women that are also key concerns for disabled women:

- gender roles
- self-image
- sexuality.

It is perhaps too early to claim that a feminist model of disability exists as such. Certainly, there is a strong feminist critique of the social model, and a strong critique of feminism by disabled women. Hansen (1995), exploring the potential for a feminist model, points out that simply 'to add disability and stir' would devalue the life experience of all women. Rather, an 'inclusive perspective' is required that would address the 'complexity, diversity and viability which is disability'. Not dissimilarly, Shakespeare (1995, p. 1) has called for 'a more reflexive sociology of disability, engaging with the feminist concept that the personal is political'.

WHERE ARE WE NOW?

As noted at the start of this chapter, there has been little cross-fertilization of ideas between the two theories that are proving most influential in the field of disability. We have noted some apparent similarity between the two, such as the emphasis on the cultural construction of disability, but this is misleading. Major differences exist, notably in normalization's identification of internal, unconscious attitudes as the principal 'problem', as opposed to the social model's concern with external material barriers. It follows that proponents of the social model reject normalization's insistence on the individual accommodating himself to social norms, striving to appear ordinary and, by implication, to 'be normal' (although it might be added that Wolfensberger has never explicitly stated that 'normality' as such is the desired goal). Nevertheless, French (1993) noted that pressures on disabled people to be 'normal', for example to use prosthetic limbs, can give rise to tremendous inefficiency and stress, while Morris (1994) adds that an assumption that disabled people *wish* to be normal, rather than just as they are, is extremely oppressive. Critical disability theory is still relatively new, however, and a range of issues continue to be debated, so this is likely to be a stimulating area of activity for some time. The fact that this is a developing subject means that occupational therapists continually need to examine their practice and be prepared to change it.

MODELS OF DISABILITY AND OCCUPATIONAL THERAPY

Occupational therapists are facing a number of challenges as the twentieth century draws to a close, not least the challenge offered by disabled people themselves. As we have seen, disabled people have come to question the dominant definitions of disability, which have been promoted by medical and other health professions, and offer alternative models (Finkelstein 1993, Oliver 1990). This has led some occupational therapists to reconsider their current understanding of disability and its impact on their work. The rest of this chapter will examine traditional and alternative perspectives on disability in the context of occupational therapy services provided to people with learning difficulties. We will begin by looking at the traditional provision of services in institutions and the community before going on to look at developments in the field.

OCCUPATIONAL THERAPY IN INSTITUTIONAL SETTINGS

Occupational therapists have a tradition of providing services to disabled people in hospital settings and in some cases continue to do so. Here, we are not referring to therapists working in acute hospital settings with people who are 'ill' and require intervention to stabilize a medical condition, but to occupational therapists working in long-stay institutions. So what do occupational therapists actually do in such settings? Case study 15.1 provides a typical example.

Occupational therapists in institutions such as Sally's typically use standardized and criterion-based assessment protocols to assess a person's physical, psychological and social development. They produce therapeutic programmes, provide equipment and make adaptations in order to maintain and improve an individual's level of functioning and to reduce 'dysfunction'.

Long-stay hospitals are often situated in remote rural areas or on the outskirts of larger cities. As a result, people generally spend the majority of their time on the hospital site, and it is assumed that all of their needs can be met there or in other specialist environments. A repertoire of therapeutic activities, such as horse-riding, hydro-therapy and multisensory environments, has developed to meet people's needs. Self-care, daily living and leisure activities are

---

Case study 15.1

Sally Wall is an occupational therapist. She works in a long-stay hospital for people with learning difficulties. Three hundred people currently live in the hospital, which has a 5-year closure plan. For the next 5 years, all of the staff's efforts will be directed towards assessing the needs of the 300 people living there, developing service specifications around these needs, looking for suitable alternative accommodation for each person and preparing people for life in the community. One of the people with whom Sally is working is called John. Sally said this about John and her work with him:

John is in his fifties now and has lived in the hospital for the past 36 years. He has learning difficulties and cerebral palsy, which has resulted in a left-sided hemiparesis. John is very institutionalized. He can do very little for himself and needs 24-hour nursing care. John cannot wash or dress himself and needs to be supervised when eating. He cannot walk without support and he uses a wheelchair when outdoors. He lives on a ward with 15 other people and shares a bedroom with seven of them. The hospital has a range of facilities on offer to residents. These include the occupational therapy department, the physiotherapy department, an activity centre that is run by nursing staff, a soft play area and a hydrotherapy pool. John spends most of his week in the hospital activity centre. While there he does a number of activities, including art work and jigsaws, and uses the computer to improve his hand–eye co-ordination and fine motor skills. He also goes to the hydrotherapy pool and comes to the occupational therapy department once a week. In the occupational therapy department, he is part of a group learning to cook simple snacks.

---

typically the target of the occupational therapist's interventions.

OCCUPATIONAL THERAPY IN THE COMMUNITY

The influence of normalization (Wolfensberger 1972), as outlined earlier in this chapter, together with the implementation of community care legislation, has led to many long-stay institutions undergoing radical reprovisioning exercises in both Britain and other countries. While some occupational therapists continue to be employed in institutions, many have moved from providing hospital-based services to providing community-based services. Community services for people with learning difficulties often use the five service accomplishments (O'Brien 1987) to inform their work. However, these are often interpreted inconsistently. Such community-based services are typically provided to people

---

Case study 15.2

Terry Evans is an occupational therapist employed in a multidisciplinary team for people with learning difficulties living in the community. The team is made up of nurses, social workers, a psychologist, a physiotherapist, a speech and language therapist and the occupational therapist. The team work mostly with people who have moved out of the local long-stay hospital into group homes. Groups of between three and six people live in these homes. Below, Terry tells us about the work he is currently undertaking with one of his 'clients'.

Tracy is 32 years old. She has severe learning difficulties and cannot communicate verbally. She has lived in a hospital for the past 20 years but has recently moved to a new home, which she shares with two other women with learning difficulties. She is very dependent on the staff at her new group home. The staff would like her to be able to do more for herself, so would like her to learn to dress herself and feed herself. They would also like her to make more use of local community facilities. Having assessed Tracy, I believe that, with a structured programme, she will be able to dress and feed herself. I have drawn up a programme for the staff to follow, which I will review with them on a monthly basis. Tracy also seems to enjoy helping staff in the kitchen. There is a course at Tracy's local college for people with learning difficulties, and one of the modules offered is catering. I have arranged a meeting between myself, Tracy and the course leader so that they can assess Tracy's suitability for the course.

---

with learning difficulties through multidisciplinary teams. This move has led occupational therapists to reconsider their role; this change is reflected in Case study 15.2.

The role of an occupational therapist in this type of service typically involves assessing the person's health and social needs, designing training programmes to encourage skills development, supporting care staff to implement training programmes and exploring opportunities for people to use their local community facilities.

THE CHANGING FACE OF OCCUPATIONAL THERAPY

The two case studies described above show that the work of the occupational therapist has changed considerably with the closure of long-stay hospitals. Services are certainly being delivered in a different environment. People are no longer encapsulated within services that are physically isolated from the rest of the population, this new physical closeness having allowed

disabled people to have a greater presence in their communities. It is now accepted that people with significant learning difficulties can live in the community and enjoy a fuller life as a result.

There have also been some changes in the type of therapeutic activity employed by occupational therapists. Self-care and daily living activities continue to be given a high priority by the therapist, however the widespread use of activities such as horse riding and hydrotherapy has increasingly been called into question. This is not to say that these activities do not have some therapeutic value for some individuals but that their widespread use is the result of the limitations placed on therapists by institutional settings rather than because they related to the individual priorities, wishes and personal interests of the people for whom they were 'prescribed'.

Community-based services tend to be provided in smaller group settings, so individual needs are more likely to be given consideration. In addition, there has been a slight shift in who provides the service. Multidisciplinary teams often rely on support workers or care assistants to provide practical hands-on training and support under their guidance.

Moving on

The work of the occupational therapist within a community-based service is certainly different from the work of an occupational therapist in an institution, but do these changes represent a new service paradigm? Those who would challenge the medical model would say that the changes have not gone far enough. As was pointed out at the beginning of this chapter, disabled people themselves are providing alternative definitions of disability. They have questioned some of the basic assumptions held by professional workers and have called for a much more fundamental shift in service provision. The assumptions that have been challenged include:

- that the 'problem' which the therapist must address is situated within the individual, and the person is the focus for intervention
- that the therapist's role is to encourage

independence, which means helping people to do as much for themselves as possible
- that professionals have expert knowledge
- that disabled people have different needs from the non-disabled population.

In both of the case studies described above, the focus of the intervention of the occupational therapist is the person. It is assumed that disability is a direct result of the person's impairment and the person therefore needs to be 'fixed' or 'cured'. The emphasis in both cases is on the person accommodating to meet the expectations of society, and the actions of the therapist are implicitly designed to make individuals more 'normal'. These assumptions have been challenged and the influence of society and the environment as sources of oppression for disabled people has been highlighted. Occupational therapists must attempt to look beyond individual explanations of disability. As a result, they must change their focus for intervention and place a greater emphasis on removing social and environmental barriers. As previously discussed, there is some disagreement within the disability movement about the adequacy of a model that looks purely at barrier removal (French 1993), but it does offer an important alternative perspective.

Redefining independence

The notion that independence is the primary aim of therapeutic intervention has been perpetuated throughout changes from hospital-based services to community-based services. Increased independence is seen by occupational therapists as a highly desirable outcome of their work. Independence in this context is defined as being able to do as much as possible for oneself. While the ability to do everyday things without being reliant on others can be liberating, disabled people have highlighted the oppressive way in which this definition can operate. Independence has been redefined by disabled people as control and self-determination (French 1994a).

For many people with learning difficulties, independence training can trap them in endless programmes from which few are allowed to

graduate. These programmes, rather than augmenting the quality of a person's life, can *become* their life. In services for people with learning difficulties, it has been assumed that the greater a person's dysfunction, the larger the residential establishment in which the person will live. The purpose of the rehabilitation process thus becomes to improve people's functioning so that they can move to gradually smaller living situations with less staff support. In reality, few people have moved to 'independent living' options, so few have gained full control over their own life. Independent living has been reformulated by disabled people to mean less about the ability of the person to live alone and more about disabled people taking full control of their lives (Morris 1993). The issue then becomes less about the person's skills and degree of readiness and more about the support they will require to live their chosen lifestyle.

Who is the expert?

Nisbet (1992) states that many assessment and planning tools currently in use in health and social services rely primarily on professional opinion and decision-making. In the past, little attention has been paid to disabled people's definition of their situation and their experience of disability. While most occupational therapists would claim to work in partnership with service users, the reality is that they have the authority to define the problem and choose the solutions. Disabled people have traditionally been passive recipients of services designed by people who do not necessarily share their values (French 1994b). It is no longer appropriate for the therapist to

---

Activity 15.4

The Canadian Occupational Performance Measure is proposed as a client-centred assessment, yet in one hospital it has been used to group people, on the basis of similar scores, as being suitable to share a group home. Would this fit with disabled people's notion of person-centredness?

Do you think that the misuse of this assessment is due to the people using it, or does the tool have design flaws such that it lends itself to misuse?

define the problem and prescribe solutions as the 'expert'. Assessment and planning tools are being developed that are more qualitative, are based on personal narratives and give primacy to the perspective of the disabled person (Falvey et al 1994, Mount 1994).

If we accept that the therapist as expert is no longer an appropriate model, we must also accept that the agenda for any work undertaken must be mutually agreed between service user and worker. Self-care and daily living skills training have traditionally been given the highest priority by occupational therapists, and the therapeutic agenda has been concerned with producing individual change. Yet people with learning difficulties are setting a new agenda and demanding that their needs for a home, a job, an income, an education, relationships, love, a feeling of belonging and control over their own lives are also met. Finkelstein (1993) calls for a partnership between service users and health and welfare professionals, and an emphasis on barrier identification and removal.

Day services for people with learning difficulties have attempted to help people with learning difficulties to find work. However, while service policies assume that a person's ability to work is determined primarily by an individual's functional abilities, only a small proportion of people will ever move out of the day service into paid employment. Instead, the emphasis needs to be placed on the ability of the workplace to modify and remove barriers (Schlaff 1993). Some occupational therapists are becoming involved in employment services that aim to alter job sites and make use of technology as a way of removing barriers (Jones 1994). Case study 15.3 demonstrates how one service has attempted to take on board some of the ideas fundamental to the social model of disability as well as taking account of the influence of the principle of normalization in services for people with learning difficulties.

CONCLUSION

Major advances have taken place in recent years in the theorization of disability, in terms

---

Case study 15.3

Jo Willis is an occupational therapist employed by an NHS community Trust. She works in a small team whose job is to support people with learning difficulties while finding work. The team is made up of a social worker, a clinical psychologist and an occupational therapist. The team use the 'five service accomplishments' (O'Brien 1987) to assess the quality of their work with individuals. Jo said this about her work with Tom, a man with learning difficulties:

Tom was the first person we were asked to support. He had attended the local adult training centre for 10 years. While there, he tended to spend most of his time in the workshop area, where he sanded wooden components that were used to make up toys and furniture. Tom had some good friends in the workshop and enjoyed chatting and joking with them as he worked. His ambition, however, was to leave the training centre one day and get a job. The staff at the training centre contacted us, with Tom's permission, to see if we could offer him any support to find a job.

We knew that it was both unrealistic and nonsensical to expect Tom to learn all of the skills required to do a particular job before he was allowed to even enter the employment market. Instead, we concentrated on identifying what Tom was good at and what his preferences were, and matching these to potential areas of employment. We then made a commitment to support Tom in whatever way he needed to find, learn and keep a job. We had to acknowledge at an early stage that there weren't any experts in this situation. Finding a job was a very new experience for Tom and a new challenge for us and employers. This was going to be a learning experience for us all.

We worked hard to make sure that Tom was fully involved in making decisions at all stages. Once we had some idea of Tom's job preferences, we approached a number of employers on his behalf and arranged some informal interviews. We expected some resistance from employers but actually, found them to be very interested in what we were doing and willing to give people a chance as long as there was support available for the new employee and themselves. Tom tried a number of short-term, unpaid job samples [work experience] before applying for and being appointed to a paid post in an office. The job samples helped Tom and the team to identify his preferences, the potential barriers that he was going to face in the workplace and his support requirements. We worked very closely with Tom, his employers and his co-workers before and during his paid job. Together, we negotiated some adjustments to Tom's job description and arranged for him to work flexible hours when his health was poor. We also came up with some simple solutions together to help Tom do the job to a high standard, for example, altering the lighting so that Tom could see more easily.

---

of identifying the limitations, and distortions, of individualistic models and the emergence of a radically different understanding of disability. The emphasis placed on the significance of material and social barriers and the resulting collective experience of oppression may, however, have led to the relative neglect of other significant factors, such as the implications of particular impairment for individuals, and also to an oversimplification of certain key concepts. The notion of 'barriers', for example, is seldom examined. It was also noted earlier that little theoretical attention has been paid to the usefulness of the social model in relation to people with learning difficulties. Although the principle of normalization and the social model of disability have not been integrated at a theoretical level, it is evident that some workers are struggling to take on board these ideas in their everyday work.

These debates and the definitions of disability that are emerging are important, not least because they have come from disabled people themselves. Occupational therapists can contribute to this process of redefinition by examining their work practices in both hospital and community settings and contributing to further control being handed back to disabled people over their own lives. As Munro & Elder-Woodward (1992, p. 41) put it:

The challenge for workers at all levels of community care is to make sure that the service user is in control of his (sic) own lifestyle and in control of the services surrounding him (sic) which are designed to support that lifestyle.

The role of the occupational therapist, if it is to take on board the perspectives of disabled people, needs to change from one of prescription and management of treatment, to making knowledge and expertise available and enabling disabled people to be aware of all their options (Craddock 1996). French (1994b) calls for services to act as a resource, as disabled people strive towards their own goals. However, there is a danger that efforts to hand back power to disabled people will be constrained while occupational therapists continue to act as 'agents of the state' (or insurance companies), i.e. employed within and accountable to bureaucratic organizations. Direct purchasing of services, including occupational therapy, by disabled people changes the relationship between disabled person and service provider. This is becoming increasingly possible as direct payments to disabled people to allow them to purchase and control their services is becoming more widely available. This is just one opportunity for further collaboration between occupational therapists and disabled people in the future.

Postscript

Since this chapter was written the World Health Organisation has announced a revision of the categories of impairment, disability and handicap. The exact nature and implications of this change, and the response of disabled people to it, are not clear at the time of going to press. The reader is advised to look out for developments in this area.

REFERENCES

Abberley P 1995 Disabling ideology in health and welfare – the case of occupational therapy. Disability and Society 10(2): 221–232

Bank-Mikkelson N 1980 Denmark. In: Flynn R J, Nitsch K E (eds) Normalisation, social integration and community services. Pro-Ed, Austin, TX

Barnes C 1991 Disabled people in Britain and discrimination: a case for anti-discrimination legislation. C Hurst, London

Begum N 1992 Disabled women and the feminist agenda. In: Hirsh H, Phoenix A, Stacey J (eds) Working out: new directions for women's studies. Falmer Press, London

Craddock J 1996 Responses of the occupational therapy profession to the perspective of the disability movement, Part 2. British Journal of Occupational Therapy 59(2): 73–78

Crow L 1995 Including all of our lives: renewing the social model of disability. Paper circulated at 'Accounting for Illness and Disability: Exploring the Divide', organized by Disability Studies Unit, University of Leeds, April 1995.

Dalley G 1988 Ideologies of caring – rethinking community and collectivism. Macmillan, London

Emerson E 1992 What is normalisation? In: Brown H, Smith H (eds) Normalisation: a reader for the nineties. Routledge, London

Falvey M A, Forest M, Pearpoint J, Rosenberg R L 1994 All my life's a circle. Using the tools: circles, maps and path. Inclusion Press, Toronto

Finch J 1984 Community care: developing non-sexist alternatives. Critical Social Policy, 9: 6–18

Finkelstein V 1980 Attitudes and disability: issues for discussions. World Rehabilitation Fund, New York

Finkelstein V 1993 Disability: a social challenge or an administrative responsibility? In: Swain J, Finkelstein V, French S, Oliver M (eds) Disabling barriers – enabling environments. Sage, London

French S 1993 Disability, impairment or something in

between? In: Swain J, Finkelstein V, French S, Oliver M (eds) Disabling barriers – enabling environments. Sage, London

French S 1994a The disabled role. In: French S (ed.) On equal terms. Working with disabled people. Butterworth Heinemann, Oxford

French S 1994b Disabled people and professional practice. In: French S (ed.) On equal terms. Working with disabled people. Butterworth Heinemann, Oxford

Gwaltney J 1970 The thrice shy: cultural accommodation to blindness and other disorders in a Mexican community. Columbia University Press, New York

Hansen N 1995 Distorted images: rethinking models of disability. Unpublished paper, Department of Applied Social Science, University of Stirling

Hevey D 1993 The tragedy principle: strategies for change in the representation of disabled people. In: Swain J, Finkelstein V, French S, Oliver M (eds) Disabling barriers – enabling environments. Sage, London

Jones C 1994 Innovative practice. In: French S (ed.) On equal terms. Working with disabled people. Butterworth Heinemann, Oxford

Morris J 1992 Personal and political: a feminist perspective on researching physical disability. Disability, Handicap and Society 7(2): 157–166

Morris J 1993 Independent lives? Community care and disabled people. Macmillan, London

Morris J 1994 Prejudice. In: Swain J, Finkelstein V, French S, Oliver M (eds) Disabling barriers – enabling environments. Sage, London

Mount B 1994 Benefits and limitations of personal futures plans. In: Bradley V J, Ashbaugh J W, Blaney B C (eds) Creating individual supports for people with developmental disabilities. Paul H Brookes, London

Munro K, Elder-Woodward J 1992 Independent living. Churchill Livingstone, Edinburgh

Nirje B 1969 The normalisation principle and its human management implications. In: Kugel R B, Wolfensberger W (eds) Changing patterns in residential services for the mentally retarded. Residential Committee on Mental Retardation, Washington DC

Nirje B 1980 The normalisation principle. In: Flynn R J, Nitsch K E (eds) Normalisation, social integration and community services. University Park Press, Baltimore

Nisbet J (ed.) 1992 Natural supports in school, at work and in the community for people with severe disabilities. Brookes, Baltimore, MD

O'Brien J 1987 A guide to lifestyle planning: using the activities catalogue to integrate services and natural support systems. In: Wilcox B W, Bellamy G T (eds) The activities catalogue: an alternative curriculum for youth and adults with severe disabilities. Brookes, Baltimore, MD

O'Brien J, Lovett H 1992 Finding a way toward everyday lives: the contribution of person centred planning. Pennsylvania Office of Mental Retardation, Pennsylvania

Oliver M 1990 The politics of disablement. Macmillan, Basingstoke

Oliver M 1993 Redefining disability: a challenge to research. In: Swain J, Finkelstein V, French S, Oliver M (eds) Disabling barriers – enabling environments. Sage, London

Oliver M 1996 Understanding disability. From theory to practice. Macmillan, London

Ryan J, Thomas F 1987 The politics of mental handicap. Free Association Books, London

Schlaff C 1993 From dependency to self advocacy: redefining disability. American Journal of Occupational Therapy 47(10): 943–948

Shakespeare T 1995 Doing it for ourselves: disability, identity and difference. Paper circulated at 'Accounting for Illness and Disability: Exploring the Divide', organized by Disability Studies Unit, University of Leeds, April 1995

Shakespeare T, Watson N 1995 The body line controversy: a new direction for disability studies? Paper circulated at Disability Studies Conference, Hull, October

Smith H, Brown H 1992 Defending community care: can normalisation do the job? British Journal of Social Work 22(6): 685–693

Whitehead S 1992 The social origins of normalisation. In: Brown H, Smith H (eds) Normalisation: a reader for the nineties. Routledge, London

Wolfensberger W 1972 The principle of normalisation in human services. National Institute on Mental Retardation, Toronto

Wolfensberger W 1983 Social role valorisation: a proposed new term for the principle of normalisation. Mental Retardation 21(6): 234–239

Glossary

Alienation the idea in marxist sociology that workers under capitalism are estranged or cut off from their product, their work, their true selves and from others.

Anomie a sense of normlessness. This concept is often associated with the work of Durkheim.

Anomie theory of deviance according to Merton, deviance occurs when the social structure precludes some groups from achieving cultural goals by legitimate means. The result is a breakdown in the social norms or anomie and a resulting pressure towards deviance.

Biomedical model belief in the objective existence of what medicine categorises as disease; which can be diagnosed treated and (generally) cured.

Class stratification a major form of social stratification in western industrial societies. It refers to the division of society into unequal groupings called social classes who differ from one another in terms of economic position and access to life chances.

Common sense 'what everyone knows', often based on naturalistic or individualistic explanations.

Culture the norms and values of a particular society; sometimes described as a way of life. Culture is learned through the process of socialisation and provides the basis for communication and cooperation between members of a society. This concept should not be confused with culture in the restricted sense of 'the arts'.

Deviance a term whose meaning varies depending on the perspective adopted. With some theories (Merton's anomie theory for example) deviance is defined as behaviour which breaks the rules. Labelling theorists, however, argue that deviance isn't simply rule-breaking but behaviour which is both seen to break the rules and which has been successfully defined as deviant.

Ethnicity a sense of belonging and loyalty to a group of common national and cultural heritage. Members of an ethnic group share descent, language, traditions, religion, and other common cultural features and experiences that distinguish them from other groups.

Ethnomethodology a perspective that directs attention to how people view order in the world, communicate that view to others and how they understand and explain social interaction.

Feminism feminist theories offer explanations for the inequalities which exist between men and women society. Traditionally there are considered to be three main perspectives; liberal feminism, radical feminism and marxist feminism.

Functionalism a development of structural-consensus theory which argues that societies should be seen as a whole made up of interrelated and interdependant parts, each part contributing to the survival of the society because of the functions it carries out. Social order and social stability are maintained through a value consensus.

Iatrogenic effects by iatrogenesis Illich means that the medical system can produce side-effects which are detrimental to the individual.

Illness iceberg the unknown extent of illness which is *not* presented to doctors and hospitals and which varies according to various perceptions and socio-economic factors

Individualistic explanations explain behaviour in terms of individuals and their particular characters, qualities and motivations without any reference to the social forces which influence their behaviour.

Labelling theory examines the way in which deviance is the outcome of an interaction between someone who is seen to break the rules and those who seek to label that person as a deviant. From this perspective there is no objective definition of deviance; deviance is behaviour which people so label.

Leisure There are various approaches to the definition of leisure; some focus on the quality of experience associated with an activity. Some see leisure as time that is not spent in work, resting or looking after oneself.

Marxism is an example of structural-conflict theory. Its basic assumption is that capitalist society is divided into two classes, the bourgeoise or ruling class who own the forces of production and the proletariat or workers who have to sell their labour to the bourgeoise in return for wages. The fact of ownership allows the bourgeoise to exploit the proletariat leading to class conflict and, ultimately, revolution.

Naturalistic explanations argue that things happen because they are somehow 'natural'.

Naturalistic explanations often include the idea that human beings, like other animals, are biologically programmed by nature to behave in particular ways.

Patriarchy The domination of women by men.

Post-modernism a collection of ideas that posits an end to modernity and is characterised by disaffection with macro-explanations, the idea of progress and the existence of objective 'truth'.

Race traditionally the notion that differences in physical characteristics between groups are indications of biological differences. Racism extends the meaning of the term to include the idea that differences in biology between physically distinct groups also mean that races differ in terms of inherited characteristics such as intelligence. A racist is someone who believes that, for biological and cultural reasons, certain physically distinct groups are superior to others. Most sociologists do not accept the idea of biologically distinct groups. Rather 'race' is a social construction, an idea that only exists within the context of social relationships and arises when one group perceives differences between itself and others which it explains in 'racial' terms.

Racialisation the social construction of different races.

Reductionism accounting for a range of phenomena in terms of a single determining factor.

Role conflict a situation where a person is confronted with incompatible role expectations, arising either from the necessity of playing two or more conflicting roles at the same time or from differing expectations within the role set.

Role making some sociologists use this term to describe the process whereby individuals create and modify roles through negotiation and individual interpretation of situations.

Role-set refers to the network of relationships which surround a particular role.

Role taking used by some sociologists to describe the process by which people undertake roles in a prescribed manner. Roles are put on or taken off like an item of clothing.

Self identity the consistent part of the self which is formed and sustained by social interaction with others

Society traditionally conceived of as a geographically bounded grouping of people sharing most norms, values and having a common identity. Note: the exact definition of what constitutes society is increasingly under debate in sociological circles.

Social constructionism is an approach concerned with how knowledge and reality are constructed in the course of everyday social interaction.

Social institution an identifiable entity which is broadly recognised and is associated with certain roles- e.g. the family, the media, higher education, etc.

Social model of disability the problems that disabled people face are seen to be as a result of the barriers created by society rather than resulting from individuals' impairments.

Social role the behaviours expected of an individual because of the social status occupied – e.g. parent, lecturer, therapist.

Social status a position or place within a social structure to which certain rights and obligations apply (see social role).

Social stratification refers to the division of society into groups which differ in terms of such things as wealth, status and power.

Sociological perspective a particular point of view or way of looking at and explaining the social world.

Sociology: the study of western industrial societies.

Status stratification refers to the division of society into a status hierarchy with each status group viewing members of their own group as equals and other groups as inferiors and superiors.

Stigma is a sign or mark which discredits a person in the eyes of others. This concept is often associated with the work of Goffman.

Structural conflict theory argues that society determines behaviour by structuring or constraining it but emphasise different factors to structural consensus theory, namely the distribution of advantage and disadvantage.

Structural-consensus theory argues that societies are held together by a value consensus which helps ensure social stability and social order.

Subcultures refers to the fact that in any society groups exist who, whilst sharing elements of the general culture, also develop their own norms and values. This difference in norms and values may be signalled by outward forms such as distinctive dress, food habits, and specific jargon that set the group apart.

Symbolic interactionism is an example of interpretive theory. Its basic premise is that people act on the basis of meanings they attach to objects and events rather than simply reacting to social forces like culture.

The family a group of persons directly linked by kin connections, the adult members of which assume responsibility for caring for children. Note the definition of the family is problematic and many sociologists have expressed dissatisfaction with a simple definition. Many different types of family have been described – e.g. the nuclear, the extended and the modified elementary.

The sociological imagination essentially means the ability to detach oneself from familiar routines, to look at them anew in order to understand the interplay between society and the individual. The sociological imagination leads to the development of sociological explanations.

Wealth refers to marketable assets, that is things that can be sold for income, and therefore means the same as property. A crucial distinction is between wealth in the form of productive property (factories etc.) and wealth as consumption property (jewellery).

Work a highly variable entity that takes on different meanings depending on the social context and the meanings assigned to it by the person and persons involved.

Work ethic the idea in capitalist society that work is a highly valued activity and that people should work hard and well.

Index